LIVING
WITH YOUR
ARTHRITIS

LIVING WITH YOUR ARTHRITIS

A Home Program for Arthritis Management

Edited by Alan L. Rosenberg, M.D.

ARCO PUBLISHING COMPANY, INC.
NEW YORK

Published by Arco Publishing Company, Inc.
219 Park Avenue South, New York, N.Y. 10003

Copyright © 1979 by Personal Health Services, Inc.

Library of Congress Cataloging in Publication Data
Main entry under title:

Living with your arthritis.

    Includes index.
    1. Arthritis.   2. Arthritics—Rehabilitation.
I. Rosenberg, Alan L.   II. Title.
RC933.P42   1978   616.7'2   77-17572
ISBN 0-668-04519-1 lib. bdg.
ISBN 0-668-04522-1 pbk.

Printed in the United States of America

Contents

Contents

Foreword

Arthritis refers to a variety of acute and chronic abnormal changes which occur in the joints of the body and the tissues in and around them. Such arthritic changes are very common, and they impair the functions of more persons than any other disease.

Although authorities have a number of theories about conditions that bring on arthritis, the cause remains obscure in several of the more disabling forms of the disease.

A specific cure is not known, but much can be done to bring relief.

Perhaps it is fortunate that the key person in a program to control arthritis and to restore joint and muscle functions is the individual who is the victim of the disease. The patient's role gains even more importance when he or she works cooperatively with and under the direction of health professionals who are specially trained and experienced in the management of patients with arthritis.

The principal purpose of this book is to supply information and direction to the arthritic person so that he or she can improve his or her condition, enjoy a more active life, and try to maintain a genuinely wholesome outlook.

After you read the contents, I suggest that you keep this volume in a prominent place in your home so that you can select certain sections to reread a number of times. Such a practice may help you to gain insight about your arthritis, to supply you with specific directions about many aspects of treatment, and to bring you needed reassurance for successfully living with your illness and mastering it.

In my many years of medical practice, profound satisfaction often came to me from witnessing patients, though troubled with a chronic illness such as arthritis, take hold of their lives, discipline their activities, and tighten up their courage. Such persons exhibited a nobility of spirit. They also often improved their physical well-being. Their constructive accomplishments were a great reward to them and an inspiration to others.

I pray that this book may help to set you on a rewarding course of management of your arthritis, assist you in coping with it, and upgrade the value of your everyday life.

F. J. L. BLASINGAME, M.D.

ABOUT DR. F. J. L. BLASINGAME

F.J.L. Blasingame, M.D. serves as President of Blasingame Associates, consultants to the health field. From 1958 to 1969, Doctor Blasingame served as Executive Vice President of the American Medical Association, and from 1937 to 1957, Doctor Blasingame was engaged in private practice. Doctor Blasingame is a member of numerous medical and health societies, including the American Medical Association, the American College of

Foreword

Surgeons, the Texas Medical Association and the Illinois State and Chicago Medical Societies. He has served as a member of the House of Delegates of the American Medical Association since 1944, as President of the Texas Medical Association 1955-56 and as a member of the Board of Trustees of the American Medical Association for eight years and Chairman of its Executive Committee for two years. He has also served for nineteen years on the Advisory Committee of the Joint Commission on the Accreditation of Hospitals and as a delegate of the American Medical Association to the World Medical Association.

Preface

The education of the arthritis patient and his family is the primary goal of this book. The many contributors to this manual, including rheumatologists, orthopedic surgeons, physical therapists, occupational therapists and social service personnel, all have important information to pass on to the arthritis sufferer. These areas of information taken together can add much to the improvement in and maintenance of function of the patient with arthritis, regardless of the severity of his disease.

The contributors to the book have also taken the position that each arthritic, armed with the necessary information about his disease must assume as much responsibility as possible for his own care. He then becomes an active partner with the medical professionals who are treating him. As an equal partner the patient can realize that he greatly influences the outcome of treatment. This knowledge should serve to motivate him to follow through on a treatment program, instead of passively placing himself in the hands of the medical professionals who are then charged with trying to help him solely through their own efforts.

Our approach to arthritis management might be considered holistic in that the recommended home program is geared to maximizing the potential of the arthritic to function on a daily basis, to preventing further disability, and to explaining his disease and the treatments he may encounter in simple terms that he can understand. We also hope to stress the interdependency between the body and mind.

I wish to acknowledge the support of Charles Jameson, Jr., President of Personal Health Services, Incorporated, of Denver, Colorado, who brought the contributors of this book together. Mr. Jameson supported and encouraged the preparation of the material in this timely book for the arthritic.

ALAN L. ROSENBERG, M.D.

ABOUT DR. ALAN L. ROSENBERG

Dr. Rosenberg obtained his undergraduate and medical degree at the University of Pittsburgh, the latter coming in 1962. After interning at the Presbyterian-University Hospital of the University of Pittsburgh he continued his training at the University of Colorado Medical Center in internal medicine and in rheumatology. His rheumatology training was under the guidance of the world famous Dr. Charley J. Smyth. After completing training with Dr. Smyth he entered private practice in Denver where he now resides and practices. In addition to his private practice in rheumatology he is an assistant clinical professor at the University of Colorado Medical Center.

Introduction

This home program for arthritis management evolved from the experiences of Personal Health Services staff in providing group therapy to arthritic patients. The Personal Health Services ten-week group therapy program consists of weekly 1½-hour sessions which include an educational presentation of various aspects of arthritis management, an exercise period, and discussion of common and individual problems. In this book, the educational presentations have been expanded to include topics which, though important to total management, may be of particular interest to only a select few of those many persons interested in learning how to live with arthritis. Suggested exercises for maintaining and increasing joint range of motion and muscle strength follow the narrative portion, and a glossary of terms and listing of sources for self-help aids and additional information will help the reader to obtain needed assistance on issues not covered in depth.

Our home program has been developed by qualified, competent health professionals including a rheumatologist, occupational and physical therapists, health educators, and others with a wide range of expertise in providing health care. It is not offered as a cure for arthritis, nor a panacea. However, the information provided can help the less severely involved arthritic to develop a home management program which can lead him to a more comfortable, satisfying way of life.

We urge anyone who suspects he has arthritis to consult a competent physician who has experience and training in diagnosing and treating rheumatological diseases. He will advise you concerning the benefits of regular exercise, medications, and other treatments proven effective in treating arthritis. We believe that any physician truly concerned with his patients' welfare will approve of following the exercises in this manual and will also welcome the educational material as a means of informing his patients of important facts about his disease.

CHAPTER ONE

Understanding Arthritis

Although it is impossible for you to know everything there is to know about your arthritis, it is important for you to understand the changes which occur within your body to upset its normal functioning. Lack of medical knowledge and training may prevent many of us from understanding scientific and medical explanations, and the terminology used by some health workers is often more baffling than a foreign language. However, we hope to present information you need in simple terms which will help you to better understand the basic mechanics of the normal joint and how it can be damaged by the disease process in arthritis. Any unfamiliar terms not explained in the text will be found in the glossary.

Let's start with a rather simple anatomy lesson. The connective tissue which supports the framework and protective covering of our bodies and its internal organs includes bones, cartilage, tendon coverings, ligaments, and the major part of the skin, joints, bursae, and blood vessels. Connective tissue plays a major role in protecting

1

the body from disease and in repairing the damage caused by injury. Each type of connective tissue has distinct physical properties which make it suitable for the function it serves.

In order to understand why the joints deteriorate, let's first look at the elegant and efficient mechanics of the normal joint. The bones of the skeleton are joined to one another in various ways, called articulations. The joints are classified according to the type of connective tissue which is involved. The three main classifications are:

1. Fibrous or synarthroses. The union is by a dense, fibrous tissue so that little or no mobility is possible. An example of this type of joint is the sacroiliac joint in the lower back.

2. Cartilagenous. In this type of joint, the space between the bones is occupied by hyaline cartilage or fibrocartilage. This type of cartilage is not so stiff as the kind found in the fibrous joints, but only a slight degree of motion is possible. The ribs are joints of this type.

3. Synovial or diarthrodial. Most of the joints of the body are this type. Nearly all of the joints in the extremities—that is, the arms and legs—are synovial joints. These joints all possess a joint cavity and are fully movable. The work demanded of this type of joint is enormous. It must be able to withstand forces many times the body weight during activity, yet move with minimal friction and maximum efficiency. It is chiefly this type of joint that is affected in joint disease. In synovial joints, the opposing surfaces of the bones are completely separated and are covered with cartilage, which is normally a milky

white, translucent, non-brittle, and homogenous substance. The ends of the bones are enveloped by a joint capsule. The outer layer of a joint capsule is composed of a dense, fibrous tissue. The inner layer consists of synovial membrane, which falls in folds surrounding the cartilage, tendons, and ligaments which pass through the joint. Normally, the synovial capsule contains a thick fluid which moistens and lubricates the joints. This synovial fluid supplies nutrition for the cartilage and plays an important part in the health of the joint. In arthritis, this synovial fluid is increased in volume and becomes thickened and yellow in color. Figure 1 shows a typical synovial joint.

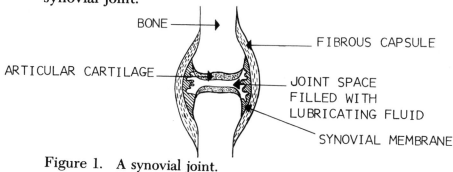

Figure 1. A synovial joint.

Each joint is designed to move in specific directions. Joint stability is largely the function of the tendons, ligaments, and muscles which normally provide enough tension and support to prevent slippage. Without this support, the cartilage can be damaged and then the joints may no longer be able to bear weight.

Diseases which involve the joints are known as rheumatic diseases. The number of rheumatic diseases which have now been identified is over 100, many of which are rarely seen. We will discuss only the three most common forms here: rheumatoid arthritis, osteoarthritis, and gout.

RHEUMATOID ARTHRITIS

Rheumatoid arthritis is the most serious because it is potentially the most destructive and crippling. Fortunately, however, only between 5 and 10 percent of all cases of arthritis are rheumatoid arthritis. The disease begins within the joints as an inflammation of the joint lining, causing an increased amount in thickened synovial fluid. There is an influx of white blood cells, which secrete chemicals which destroy the tissue and cartilage. A mantle of tissue or pannus eats its way through the cartilage and even through the bone ends. Finally, scar tissue is transformed into tissue which not only interferes with joint mobility, but which eventually may cause spontaneous fusion of the joint. This fusion makes further movement of the joint impossible. The loss of cartilage and the weakening of tendons, ligaments, and other supportive structures results in instability and partial dislocation of the joint. Unlike osteoarthritis, rheumatoid arthritis may affect the entire body. Other complications affecting organs such as the lungs, heart, and eyes may impose a more serious threat than the joint disability. Figure 2 shows the course of rheumatoid arthritis in a joint.

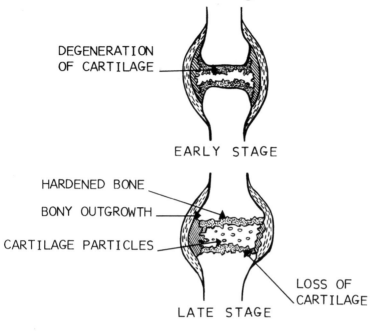

DEGENERATION
OF CARTILAGE

EARLY STAGE

HARDENED BONE

BONY OUTGROWTH

CARTILAGE PARTICLES

LOSS OF
CARTILAGE

LATE STAGE

Figure 2. The course of rheumatoid arthritis in a
joint.

The cause of rheumatoid arthritis is unknown, but
several theories have been advanced. Among them are:

1. Autoimmune response; that is, a defense mechanism reaction or an allergy to one's own tissue
2. A viral infection
3. A combination of the first two; that is, the infection
is so persistent that the body builds up antibodies against
its own tissue.

5

Final proof of any of these theories is not yet in, and an urgent need for further research to find the cause remains.

The course and severity of the disease varies widely among patients, and is characterized by a tendency toward alternating periods of spontaneous remission and flare-up. This means that it seems to go away by itself—one out of ten cases do remit—and then it returns. Because symptoms may appear and then subside at intervals ranging from days to years, and attacks may be sudden or insidious and range from mild to severe, medical diagnosis is often delayed. These "ups and downs" have no set pattern, but gradually the attacks become more severe and closer together and the disease becomes chronic and progressive. It then can no longer be ignored.

Prompt diagnosis and treatment are imperative, but an accurate evaluation to exclude other possibilities is difficult. A complete and careful physical examination utilizing blood, urine, and joint fluid tests together with X-rays may be used. The findings are then put together to draw a comprehensive picture of the patient's condition and a diagnosis is made.

Persons with rheumatoid arthritis will typically have aching and stiffness, especially in the morning, and pain, heat, swelling, and redness of the involved joints. Rheumatoid arthritis often affects both members of the paired parts of the body; that is, both knees or hands may be involved. In chronic rheumatoid arthritis, there is increasingly serious and permanent disturbance of joint function, muscular weakness followed by wasting away of the muscles, erosion of cartilage, and small, firm, round-

6

ed masses or nodules may form under the skin. About 75 percent of all patients with rheumatoid arthritis show an elevated level of what is called rheumatoid factor in the blood. This elevated level of rheumatoid factor is found by laboratory blood tests, which also may reveal an increased white blood cell count during an acute flare-up, low-grade anemia, increased sedimentation rate, and elevated gammaglobulin level. If these tests are made, your physician will no doubt explain their significance to you and their importance in diagnosing rheumatoid arthritis. Fatigue, fever, and weight loss may also be symptoms. Involvement of the internal organs such as the lining of the heart (pericarditis), lungs (pleuritis), irritation of the nerves (neuritis), or irritation of the lining of the eye (scleritis), are examples of complications observed in patients with rheumatoid arthritis that is more severe and longer in duration.

There is no cure for rheumatoid arthritis. There is no foolproof way to arrest the disease or produce a remission. And there is no evidence that the more potent drugs can relieve symptoms fully and regularly. On the other hand, there *is* ample evidence that a treatment program consisting of rest, medication, physical and occupational therapy, and possibly surgery, all as indicated during various stages of the disease, should be followed. As you can see, the physician must assess many factors in order to decide the course of action to be taken in controlling rheumatoid arthritis. Among these factors are: 1) duration of the disease, 2) presence of manifestations or complications, 3) degree of disease activity, 4) joint status, and 5) age, sex, and life style of the patient. The disease is complex and the combination of measures dealing with it must be continued faithfully over a long period.

As a rule, women are affected more often than men, by a three-to-one ratio. The adult form of rheumatoid arthritis usually strikes the age group under forty, but it may begin at any age. When children under sixteen years of age are involved, it is referred to as juvenile rheumatoid arthritis, which usually strikes most children between 2-5 and 9-12 years of age. About 70 percent of these young patients regain normal or near normal joint function by adulthood.

About three-fourths of the patients who have had symptoms of rheumatoid arthritis for less than one year will improve, and 15-20 percent may show complete remission. What is the outlook for the long-term patient? Observations extending over a period of many years show that only 10 percent of all patients eventually become incapacitated; that is, they cannot function without almost total care.

OSTEOARTHRITIS

Now let's look at another member of the arthritis family, osteoarthritis. What happens when joints age? As you know, in a normal joint, the surfaces slide smoothly in movement. Repeated use in weight-bearing and repeated impact or injury can cause the mechanical parts of the joint to wear out as a person gets older. The cartilage then becomes rough and frayed, and eventually may be worn off. Changes also occur in the underlying bone. Irregular and sometimes very large spurs of new bone covered by

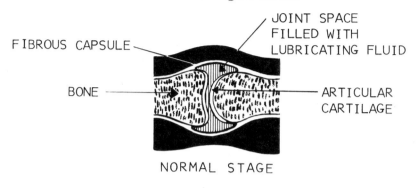

FIBROUS CAPSULE

JOINT SPACE
FILLED WITH
LUBRICATING FLUID

BONE

ARTICULAR
CARTILAGE

NORMAL STAGE

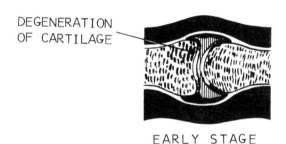

DEGENERATION
OF CARTILAGE

EARLY STAGE

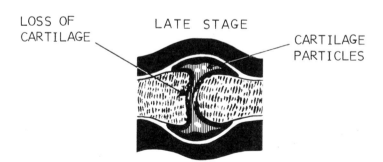

LOSS OF
CARTILAGE

LATE STAGE

CARTILAGE
PARTICLES

Figure 3. Osteoarthritis.

9

cartilage, which are known as osteophytes, form at the joint margins and places where ligaments and muscles are attached. These osteophytes restrict or eventually prevent normal motion. Broken-off chips of the "spurs" or "joint mice" may appear in the joint cavity. This common, non-inflammatory, progressive disorder of the movable joints is also referred to as degenerative joint disease. Of the fifty or so terms used to describe this condition, osteoarthritis remains the most popular, and we will use these two terms interchangeably.

Your doctor may tell you that you have either "primary" or "secondary" osteoarthritis. Primary osteoarthritis is the result of years of wear and tear on the joints. It is the most common form of arthritis, affecting over forty million Americans, and appears to be an inherent part of the aging process. However, it is by no means restricted to the elderly. It may be seen relatively early in life, although some people live quite long without any apparent trouble with it.

A variety of factors in addition to aging may determine the pace of cartilage degeneration and the subsequent progression of the disease. Secondary degenerative joint disease may occur as a result of one of the following:

1. An injury to a specific joint.
2. Excessive strains and stresses on joints.
3. Developmental structural abnormalities.
4. Metabolic disturbances.
5. Repeated joint hemorrhage.
6. Neurological disorders.
7. Hereditary predisposition.

Understanding Arthritis

The most common symptom of degenerative joint disease is pain. This pain occurs in the joints particularly upon motion or weight-bearing, and may be accompanied by stiffness after periods of rest. Pain may be severe or mild, constant or intermittent, and increased pain may be noticed in bad weather. Weakness and spasm of the surrounding muscles with loss of joint motion, which eventually changes the alignment and causes deformity, is the next most common complaint. There may be grating when the joint is moved. Often this grating can be heard or felt, though in itself it causes little pain. The joint may be tender and swollen, but the synoviam is not inflamed. Fever, weight loss, or a general feeling of illness are not common symptoms of osteoarthritis. The white blood count, sedimentation rate, and serum proteins are usually normal, and the blood test for the rheumatoid factor is negative. In diagnosing osteoarthritis, the physician takes these negative laboratory findings into account, along with the results of a physical examination, a patient history, and X-rays.

When we hear the term "arthritis" we immediately think of a generalized disease which has the potential to totally incapacitate. Fortunately, however, osteoarthritis is usually confined to only a few joints. The bilateral or symmetrical pattern of involvement of the joints which is common in rheumatoid arthritis is generally not found in osteoarthritis.

How do you treat osteoarthritis? As in rheumatoid arthritis, you should continue a medically supervised treatment program aimed at relief of pain and maintenance of joint function. Preventative measures should be taken to avoid disability and disease progression. Rest and support, heat or cold, exercise, traction, and weight reduction can be helpful. The moderate use of anti-inflammatory drugs such as aspirin and an occasional injection of corticosteroids into the affected joints may be prescribed. Surgical procedures are sometimes necessary for relief of persistent pain and correction of serious deformity.

GOUT

Now let's turn our attention to the third member of the arthritis family, gout. In the mid-1800's Sir Alfred Baring Garrod, a young physician in England who is recognized as "The Father of Modern Rheumatology," presented his masterful clinical account of gout. His research on the relationship between uric acid and gout forms the basis of our modern understanding of this disease.

This acutely painful form of arthritis claims at least a million victims in the United States, which makes it far more common than generally believed. Almost 90 percent of the patients are men between thirty and fifty years of age. Gout in women usually begins in the post-menopausal period, after about age fifty.

In contrast to most other types of arthritis, the onset of joint inflammation in gout is very rapid, with severe pain and swelling within a few hours. In three out of four cases, the great or big toe is the first part of the body affected. Later, however, it may affect any joint in the arms or legs. The victim usually describes the attack as one of such intense, violent pain that he cannot bear even the weight of the bedsheet or the slightest movement of his toe. There is considerable swelling, redness, and fever, and when this inflammation subsides, the overlying skin may peel off. Untreated attacks of gout may last for several days or several weeks. The interval between attacks is usually entirely free of symptoms. Many years may pass between the first and second episodes, but as the years go by, attacks tend to become more frequent, more severe, involve more than one joint, and last longer.

The formation and removal of uric acid is the problem in this form of arthritis. All patients with gout, unless treated, have an increased uric acid level. This condition is known as hyperuricemia. This means that uric acid, which is a normal body substance, is either over-produced or produced faster than the body can eliminate it. Needle-like uric acid crystals are found in the joint fluid. Some years after the initial attack, masses of uric acid known as tophi, or "articulation badges," appear in and around the joints, in the kidneys, and under the skin of the hands, heels, and elbows. Tophi are distinguished from rheumatoid nodules by their crystal-like formation and chalky-white content, and they are harder, larger, more irregular in shape, and may ulcerate and drain. More frequent and severe attacks of gout produce additional deposits. Erosion of cartilage and bone and eventually joint deformity follow.

Primary gout is the term applied to cases in which hyperuricemia results from an inherited error of metabolism or body chemistry. For unexplained reasons, there is an over-production and/or retention of uric acid. A great majority of the patients with gout seem to have a familial tendency toward the disease. In secondary gout, hyperuricemia is directly related to other diseases, environmental disorders, or the use of certain medications such as diuretic pills which are used to decrease body fluid and lower blood pressure.

The classic picture of King Henry VIII gorging himself on rich food and drink while his gouty foot is propped on a stool is one we might recall from history class. For a long time now, this image has associated excessive indulgence in food and drink with gout. It is easy to see that people who "eat well" produce more uric acid, and the consumption of large amounts of alcohol can also interfere with the normal excretion of uric acid. In similar fashion, prolonged, severe fasting can induce hyperuricemia and restrict kidney excretion of uric acid. With drug therapy, dietary management has become less important; however, excess weight should be avoided and foods high in purine, which is the base for forming uric acid, should not be eaten. Some foods high in purine are kidneys, liver, sweetbreads, sardines, and anchovies.

The two chief objectives in treatment of gout are to reduce the uric acid in the system to tolerable levels and to control and prevent further attacks. With the medications currently available, such as colchicine, phenylbutazone, and allopurinol, it is possible to achieve both of these objectives and maintain normal levels of uric acid in most gouty arthritis sufferers. In comparison to other types of arthritis, gout can almost always be controlled by faithfully following a program of medication. Because medication controls rather than cures the disease, the medication must be continued for life.

Understanding Arthritis

Diseases of the joints have been observed in the skeletal remains of Neanderthal man from 40,000 B.C. and in the fossil dinosaur skeletons from 200,000 B.C. You might think that a disease so ancient and widespread as arthritis would by now be completely understood. Yet, a society which has sent men to the moon and conquered space is still struggling to find solutions to the numerous mysteries of the complex list of rheumatic diseases. Hopefully, the new knowledge and discoveries of research and investigation are advancing us to the point where a major breakthrough can be expected to lead us to conquering arthritis.

CHAPTER TWO

Posture, Exercise, and Rest

Understanding the importance of posture, exercise, and rest is basic to developing good habits which can help you live more comfortably with your arthritis. In learning more about these fundamental aspects of good health, you will become aware of how some simple changes in your daily habits can make a great deal of difference in how you feel. The ultimate goal is to develop a daily program which can help maintain and even increase your ability to function better with less fatigue, pain, and fear of further damaging your arthritic joints.

First, let's consider posture and positioning, because the way you stand, sit, and lie during exercise and rest is very important. For each of us, correct posture is vital to good health. For the *arthritic*, the practice of good body mechanics is imperative. Your tendency to assume positions in which painful joints are most comfortable can either cause or lead to more serious problems and deformities.

Correct posture in standing is with the head held tall, shoulders straight and slightly back, abdomen tucked in, and the hips and knees straight. You should feel natural and comfortably at ease; don't exaggerate the idea of holding your body in proper alignment to the point where you feel and look stiff and uncomfortable. Even though the proper posture may feel strange at first, you will soon become accustomed to it and, with practice, will assume good posture automatically. Harmful deviations include holding the head forward at the neck, stooped shoulders, "swayback," bent hips or knees, and turned-in ankles. In walking you should maintain the correct standing position, with you arms hanging naturally at your sides. In this position, your arms are free to help you balance. Do not carry heavy packages hanging at your sides, or use shoulder-strap handbags. You must remember to always distribute your weight equally on both feet, shifting your weight from one side to the other as smoothly as possible. If you feel unsteady, you may want to separate your feet a few more inches to provide better balance. If your ankles tend to swell after periods of standing or walking, you will feel better if you lie down and elevate them higher than your head for at least thirty minutes. Figures 4a, b, and c show correct and incorrect standing posture.

In bending to reach the floor, bend the hips and knees slightly, keeping the back straight. *Never* bend at the back or lift in this position. And if you should consider turning while in this squat position, *don't!* It is safer to stand up again, turn your body, and repeat the squat to the other side. This method of bending can spare a lot of stress and strain to the middle and low regions of the back.

Sitting is usually more comfortable than standing. If you sit for long periods, you will be more comfortable in a

17

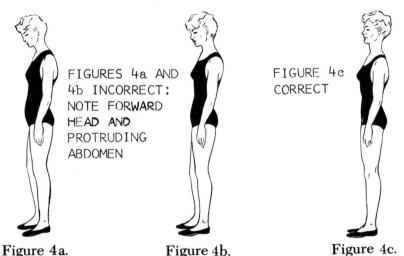

FIGURES 4a AND
4b INCORRECT:
NOTE FORWARD
HEAD AND
PROTRUDING
ABDOMEN

FIGURE 4c
CORRECT

Figure 4a.   Figure 4b.   Figure 4c.

good chair with a firm seat, a back support with a slight curve to support the lumbar or lower area of your back, and arm rests to support your arms and hands. If you are engaged in some activity at a table or desk, the chair should be placed so that you do not have to strain or slump to reach the work surface. Your legs should not be crossed and your feet should be flat on the floor or on a stool. The same principles of good posture—i.e., head up, shoulders straight, abdomen in—should be applied while sitting. If you must lean forward, lean from the waist. Do *not* sit for long periods of time without getting up and moving about. Changing positions frequently is a must for persons with arthritis. Figure 5 shows correct sitting posture, and Figure 6 illustrates the proper way to lift objects from the floor.

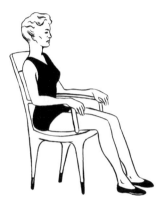

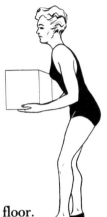

Figure 5. Correct sitting posture.

Figure 6. Proper way to lift objects from floor.

When resting or sleeping, it is important that you have a good, firm mattress. If your mattress sags, a bedboard or piece of plywood at least one-half inch thick may be placed between the mattress and the springs. The height of your bed should be such that you can get off and on easily. A bed which is too low can be raised by placing blocks of wood under the legs.

A pillow may be used under your head, but it should be placed so that it supports your shoulder blades and not just pushes your neck forward. *Never* use pillows to bend your knees. During long periods of confinement, or if you have arthritis of the back, it may be necessary to vary your position from lying on your back. Alternate positions such as lying on your side for short intervals or even lying on your stomach with your feet extended over the edge of the

19

bed may be useful. By the way, the latter position is an excellent way to stretch the long muscles in the hips and knees, which often become contracted. In some cases, positioning by use of footboards, sandbags, and splints may be beneficial. A physical therapist can help you in this matter if your physician recommends that you use such devices. Figure 7 shows correct back-lying position and Figure 8 shows how footboards and other devices can be used.

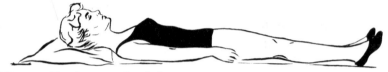

Figure 7. Correct back-lying position.

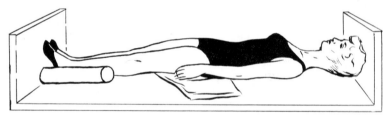

Figure 8. Use of footboards and other devices.

Analyze your posture as it is now, or ask a friend or neighbor to help you in the evaluation. Where you can correct bad habits, do so, and try to apply these principles we have given you. Whether you are resting or doing exercises, good posture will pay off with better results and less strain on your joints.

We most frequently associate "rest" with the time spent sleeping at night. Sleep is a universal need which requires no further discussion; however, the requirements for rest for the chronically ill person differ from those of a healthy individual. You may find that it takes longer and demands more of your energy to accomplish the amount of work which you did with ease when in better health. Fatigue which resulted from prolonged and excessive exertion when you were younger and more robust may now come after a fifteen-minute walk, preparing dinner, or ten minutes of exercise. It is important for you to recognize that this increased discomfort and decreased efficiency signals your body's need for a brief rest. It may be frustrating to slow down, but you will experience less stress if you alternate your physical and mental activities throughout the day. Pain and fatigue associated with arthritis is a deterrent to your ability to relax, so it is helpful to work out a program of medication as needed combined with rest periods and other techniques which can help you learn to relax. More will be said about relaxation and pain control later.

Now, just how can you determine what a balanced rest-exercise program is? This will vary for each person. No two people have the same requirements for rest or the identical tolerance for exercise. You will have to determine your own requirements and limits. The type, duration, and frequency of exercise you will need will depend upon many factors. The first is the involvement and severity of your arthritis. Second, if you have been fairly active physically, you can undoubtedly tolerate more exercise than a person who has engaged in very restricted or no activity. Third, if you suffer from another illness such as heart disease, respiratory problems, or similar chronic or acute conditions, your doctor will no doubt advise you to limit your activities somewhat. All these considerations will affect your ability to perform exercises such as the ones we recommend, and you should follow your physician's advice. We urge you to know your limitations and be aware of any ill effects you may experience either during or after exercising.

The dictionary defines exercise as "the performance of physical activity for the improvement of health or correction of deformity." We all need exercise in some form to maintain normal body functions. Properly performed, exercise can help increase your range of motion, decrease decalcification of bone to some degree, prevent muscle wasting, and build up muscle strength. You are not expected to train the way an athlete does for competition, nor to reach the level of performance of a young, healthy person at the peak of physical condition. However, a regular program of exercise can improve your ability to perform your daily activities. Another beneficial effect of exercise is the increased circulation of lymph and blood, which can be especially helpful in relieving pain in the joints and connective tissue and also in relieving swelling.

In arthritis, we are concerned with exercises which have the specific purpose of moving the joints by voluntary contractions and relaxations of the muscles involved. Many forms of exercise can be used to achieve this objective. Exercise can be classified as passive, active-passive, active, resistive, and static.

In passive exercise, the motion is initiated and carried through by another person or force. That is, the patient who is unable to perform on his own at all receives the movement from another's action. If the person is able to move or contract a muscle but needs assistance to complete the action, this is called active-assistive exercise. Active exercise is when the patient contracts and relaxes his muscles and thus moves parts of his body without assistance from another. When any force or resistance is applied against the motion of the body part, the resulting exercise is known as resistive exercise. This type of exercise is used to build muscle strength and bulk. The last type, static, is simply a sustained tightening or "setting" of the muscle without motion.

Exercises also may be classified into four major categories according to the results desired: 1) range of motion, 2) stretching, 3) strengthening, and 4) functional.

Range of motion exercises. The place where the union between two or more bones of the body occurs is called a joint. At this union there is a specific amount of movement performed by the muscles which are attached to the bones. This movement in various directions is referred to as range of motion. Examples are range of motion of the hip, which is a ball and socket joint; the knee, which is a hinge joint; and the neck. You should learn how far your joints can move normally and always exercise the body part to the fullest range, limited only by pain, in order to maintain the normal range and to increase it where it has been impaired.

Stretching exercises. Stretching is done to relieve tightness or stiffness in the tendons and muscles surrounding a joint. When a joint is not used because of pain, the muscles that control that joint are inactive. This disuse causes decreased flexibility and spasm or cramping, which can be relieved by a mild stretching action.

Examples are tightness or pain in the calf and the hamstrings. Stretching must be done very carefully and should not be done for a joint which has become spontaneously or surgically fused.

Strengthening exercises. These are used to increase muscle power and work ability. The greater the demand placed upon the muscle, the greater the number of muscle fibers used for the contraction. Strength is built up by increasing the frequency of the action, by the duration of the contraction, and/or by the amount of resistance applied. This resistance can be external. For example, another person can push against the part being exercised or you can work against gravity or weights. The force can also be internal, as in isometric exercise. This form of "muscle setting" requires minimal joint movement while increasing strength. Examples are tightening the abdominal or thigh muscles. When you cannot move inflamed joints, this form of exercise is particularly helpful.

Functional Exercise. This form of exercise is actually the ultimate goal of the types of exercises previously discussed. What you really want to achieve is the ability to function independently in performing essential personal and household tasks such as combing your hair, buttoning your clothes, shaving, preparing dinner, and driving the car. Some ways you can use certain activities, skills, hobbies, and recreational interests for beneficial exercise are: playing the piano, for hand exercise; swimming, for general exercise and endurance; and walking, to exercise the legs and improve circulation. If you already have

24

functional deficits, you may find it necessary to learn a new way to accomplish some desired tasks.

Now you know all about posture, rest, and exercise, but before you start exercising, let's summarize a few special and very important rules. We stress that these rules are very important because unless you heed them you may end up aching and discouraged.

Rule 1. You are an individual. Your arthritis is not the same as that of anyone else. Therefore, what you do in an exercise program will not be the same as what another person may do. Please do not compare your medications, how much exercise or rest you need, or home remedies. Your only competition is your arthritis! Set your goals and adapt our program to your needs. Then make up your mind to stick to that program faithfully.

Rule 2. Start exercising slowly and carefully. It is usually safe to move the joint in each direction three to five times and very gradually increase as your tolerance permits. The actions should be performed smoothly, avoiding sudden, jerky, and rapid movements.

Rule 3. Most exercise programs can be performed in two sessions of twenty to thirty minutes daily. However, we very strongly believe that if your scheduling permits, you will get better results with frequent short periods of exercise than you will by several long sessions. Plan your entire daily routine around alternate periods of activity and rest.

Rule 4. When your illness is acute or you have a "flare-up," you will have to ease up and may require assistance in performing a limited amount of activity.

25

Posture, Exercise, and Rest

Your need for rest, good posture, and proper positioning is even greater during this time. We caution you to resist the temptation to over-exert during this time. On the other hand, when you feel relatively little pain, you can stress strengthening and endurance exercises. Isometric exercises can be beneficial during periods you are not feeling as well as usual, and can be performed even while sitting or lying in bed.

Rule 5. You may, and probably will, experience increased pain after exercising, especially when you start too vigorously. Some discomfort is to be expected, but if it lasts over a period of one hour, decrease the amount of exercise. Many persons exercise for seven to ten days without ill effects, then experience pain and tiredness for a day or two. This may discourage you, but it will soon pass and you will find that you have an increased capacity for exercise after these episodes. Don't give up!

Rule 6. Finally, do not expect too much too soon! Try to accept each day as a step nearer to your individual goal.

Rule 7. Start today.

The Personal Health Services Home Program exercises start on page 168.

CHAPTER THREE

The Use of Physical Therapy Modalities in Arthritis Treatment

There is no question that the greatest contribution made by physical therapy to the arthritic is in the area of proper exercising, which aims at the maintenance and restoration of mechanical function and alignment of the joints. We know, however, that recurrent attack of pain can keep you from carrying out an exercise program. Your physician has most likely prescribed anti-inflammatory and analgesic medications to help control your pain. In addition, there are physical therapy measures, or modalities, which can help you to move more freely and relieve some of the bothersome aches and pains due to degenerative joint disease. In this chapter we shall discuss the use of these physical therapy modalities in arthritis treatment because it is important for you to know what is available and how to apply some of the techniques at home.

Physical Therapy Modalities

Treatment by means of physical agents such as light, heat, cold, exercise, water, electricity, and mechanical agents is known as physical therapy. These measures have been known and used in treating and curing ailments since ancient times, yet it has taken the medical profession many years to truly accept their value. However, with increased research and verification of its beneficial effects on the body, physical therapy has become an integral part of accepted medical treatment. Most physicians recognize that physical therapy measures which are applied to the surfaces of the body can make an effective contribution to arthritis management, especially when followed by range of motion exercises. Note that we said contribution, not cure! We present these modalities as aids to help you be more active and more comfortable in spite of having arthritis. You should not use any of these measures we will describe without prior consultation with and approval of your doctor. As with your medication, he will advise you regarding your individual needs and recommend the physical therapy measures you can safely use to keep your arthritis under control and help you to feel better. What might be beneficial for one patient may be totally wrong for another. It may sound repetitious, but you must let your doctor decide what is best for you. If he feels that you should use applications of heat and cold, for example, the following information will help you to understand some of the ways and means to do this at home.

An analgesic is an agent which helps to relieve pain. Thermotherapy, or heat, is the oldest form of analgesic. Early man discovered that sunlight warmed his body and made him feel good. He used hot packs of mud or herbs to relieve his sore muscles and used spas for their supposed curative powers. In modern times we can enjoy the luxury of a warm bath following a day of vigorous activity. What are some of the effects of heat on the body that produce these good feelings? There is an increase in temperature of the area resulting from increased circulation and metabolic rate. The over-all benefit that an arthritic will obtain is relief of pain and muscle spasm, which will allow greater mobility of the joint. This is especially desirable before exercise. Also, because of its analgesic and sedative or calming effects, heat can be helpful as an aid to more complete relaxation following exercise.

Remember that individual considerations will affect whether or not certain treatments should be used. For example, in the acute inflammatory stage, the application of heat to the affected joint may aggravate your symptoms or cause increased swelling or trauma, and so should not be applied. Other contraindications include very young or very old persons, both of whom usually have less tolerance for temperature extremes. Therefore, you must be cautious not to apply too much heat for too long a period. Some patients feel that if a little heat is good, a lot will be that much better, but this is a good way to get burned. Since impaired circulation and decreased sensation usually accompany aging, you must carefully determine your individual tolerance.

Close attention must be given to the intensity and duration of the application. Any heat application should make you feel comfortably warmed and should be applied while you are in a relaxed position. In general, the desired effects are obtained in about twenty minutes; the margin of safety can vary a few minutes either way. The only way to know how frequently heat is needed is by observing the results of its use. Unlike medication, heat is an external measure and can, without harmful effects, be used two or three times daily or two or three times a week. It should be discontinued if you experience increased or prolonged pain after usage. However, if you are uncertain of the benefits received, you may want to stop for a while to see if the application of heat has made any difference. You may wish to change to a different form of heat after comparing the reactions from each type. Basically, there are two types of heat, moist and dry. One may work better for you than the other, or you may want to try alternating them.

Hydrotherapy, or water baths, includes therapeutic pools, the Hubbard Tub, which is found in hospitals and clinics, whirlpools of various sizes and shapes, hot and cold contrast tubs, and the home bath tub. The use of a warm pool, Hubbard Tub, or whirlpool is ideal for providing general heat while allowing you to perform range of motion exercises. Weakened and painful joints can be easily moved in the water, which supports the weight of the body. Again, the temperature should be comfortably warm, ranging from body temperature 98.6° to 108° for localized areas. Since hydrotherapy is fatiguing, your general condition should be considered in regulating the temperature of the water and the duration of the treatment, which usually is twenty to thirty minutes. Although few of us have whirlpool or therapy pools in our homes, almost everyone has a bath tub. You can use it as a therapeutic device, controlling the temperature and duration to accomplish the best results for your condition. A thermometer can assure your using water of the proper temperature and a timer will help you regulate the duration. You must be extremely careful in getting in and out of the tub in order to avoid a fall, which certainly will not help your arthritis!

Moist heat can be applied locally in the form of hydrocollator packs or turkish towel compresses. The hydrocollator pack consists of a siliate gel in a cotton bag. These bags are heated in a hot water bath (160°-175°), removed and wrapped in terry cloth covers, then applied to the painful area for twenty minutes. These packs can be purchased for home use from a medical supply company and heated in a pan of water on the stove. Also, some electric heating pads can be used safely with moisture. Just make sure you check the instructions on the pad before using it that way. Use hot packs, electric pads, and hot water bottles carefully. Serious burns can result if you do not limit the time and intensity of application.

Immersion of the arms or legs in hot and cold water alternately is known as contrast bath. This procedure is effective in reducing swelling. The patient places his arms and/or legs in hot water (110°) for three minutes, then in cold water (60°) for one minute, alternating the cycle for a total of twenty to thirty minutes.

The use of wax, melted to 126° to make a hot paraffin bath, is often a preferred method of applying heat to the hands, although not limited to that area. The technique of dipping until a "glove" of one-fourth to one-half inch thickness is formed, is described in detail at the end of this chapter, so we will not go into detail here. Wax is highly flammable, so it must be handled with extreme caution, following the written guidelines exactly.

The application of dry heat through a process known as radiation is accomplished by using luminous and infra-red lamps and household electric heaters. In a hospital or clinic physical therapy department, the intensity is carefully controlled by the distance from the bulb or coil to the skin surface. Since there is an increased danger of blistering and "hot spots" with dry heat, we want to stress a few precautions:

1. Check safety features very carefully before purchasing commercial lamps. Bulbs can explode while in use, so they should always have a protective screen cover.
2. Do not rub skin with ointments prior to heat application.
3. Carefully adjust the distance and intensity as specified on a particular product.
4. Finally, but *most* important, guard against falling asleep while under any heat lamp or any source of external heat. Many burns occur this way. An inexpensive timer with an alarm can prevent overexposure.

The physiological effects of dry heat do not differ much from those of moist heat, and the frequency and duration of treatment should be controlled by your tolerance. One item which is not classified as therapy equipment, but which can be utilized at home very easily, is the electric blanket. It has become a constant nighttime companion of many arthritics who find its gentle warming useful in relieving the usual morning stiffness. By removing the weight of heavy blankets on weakened, painful joints, you lessen the chances of deformity and obtain relief with the heat it provides.

A deeper penetration and treatment of a more localized area can be achieved by use of diathermy and ultrasound machines. They are not adaptable for home use. Since they should be operated by skilled technicians, our only purpose in including them is to mention them as an additional source of heat. There is still a difference in medical opinion regarding their effectiveness in treating arthritis. While effective in treating some musculoskeletal diseases such as bursitis, myositis, and fibrositis, ultrasound and diathermy should not be used for all forms of arthritis. Allow your doctor to advise you on their use.

Some patients benefit from heat application, while others seem to obtain greater relief with the use of cold. You may receive more relief from heat during one stage of your illness, while at another time, cold may help you more. Occasionally they can be used in combination. In acutely inflamed rheumatic joints, the anesthetic effect of cold helps to deaden the pain by desensitizing the nerve endings. Locally, cold restricts the blood flow, which is why it is used on an injury or bruise to stop the bleeding. Cold also causes a decrease in cellular activity. In severe muscle spasm and following surgical repair of an arthritic joint, the local application of cold may be better than heat because of the anesthetic effect as well as the decreased blood flow.

33

Physical Therapy Modalities

We have already mentioned hot and cold contrast in discussing thermotherapy techniques. The ice pack, ice bag, and turkish towels soaked in ice water, then wrung out and applied to the desired area for 15-20 minutes, are easy methods of cold application. In recent years an ice rub or massage has gained in popularity.

The use of massage for relief of pain and suffering dates back to antiquity. Massage is a scientific rubbing and manipulation of the skin and soft tissues of the body. Following bathing in the hot mineral spas or in hot mud, it was a common practice to anoint the body with oils and to stroke the skin and tissues. The gentle stroking induced muscular relaxation, while the mechanical reaction of rapid or deep stroking caused a contraction of the muscles. When properly done by a trained therapist, massage can be useful in arthritis therapy. A good massage can: 1) dilate or enlarge the superficial blood vessels, which leads to better blood circulation, 2) stimulate sensory nerve endings, 3) reduce swelling, 4) help carry off waste products, 5) decrease muscle spasm, 6) loosen and stretch tendons and ligaments, 7) dissolve soft adhesions, 8) act as a sedative. However, it is *not* true that a vigorous massage will reduce fat or take off inches, except for the masseuse!

A variety of movements is used in massage: effleurage (stroking), friction, petrissage (kneading), percussion (tapotement), compression, and vibration. Experience and a skillful sense of touch will help the therapist to determine the correct pressure and to combine these movements to produce the desired effects. As you can see, do-it-yourself massage is not advised.

34

Physical Therapy Modalities

Heat is usually applied before massage, and the patient is placed in a position which will help him to relax. Tenseness, discomfort, and chilling can reduce the beneficial effects of massage. Some pointers to remember:

1. Painful and swollen joints should never be massaged. A light stroking may be done around adjacent areas, however.
2. Massage used in arthritis should never produce pain which lasts for several hours.
3. Disregard claims made by commercial lubricants. Although they are counterirritants and produce a warm feeling, it is the massage that produces the desired effects, and any lubricant is satisfactory.
4. If there is malignancy, phlebitis, dermatitis, osteomyelitis, or any other illness, your doctor will not recommend massage.

Another measure which may be utilized in some forms of cervical or lumbar arthritis is traction. This is a force or system of forces applied to the body along its length in such a manner as to pull or separate the joint spaces. Traction is frequently used in arthritis on the hip, knee, elbow, and fingers. Reasons for its use are: 1) to produce rest by immobilization, 2) to overcome muscle spasm, and 3) to relieve compression by separating bony surfaces. Traction may be used continuously or intermittently, and may be applied with the patient in a sitting or lying position. Traction tables and units are standard equipment in most hospital or clinic physical therapy departments, but there are many ways to improvise with ropes, weights, and sandbags at home. Perhaps you are already familiar with the Sayre traction unit or head halter, which is commonly prescribed for home use. If your physician recommends the use of traction at home, he may direct you to a physical therapist who will provide guidance and supervision so that you can use it at home with the maximum possible benefit.

We are not suggesting that you try everything we have mentioned. On the contrary, *do not try anything* until you have the approval of your doctor, who can advise you on the use of these physical therapy measures.

On the following pages you will find instructions on the use of some of the techniques mentioned. These have been adapted for easy use in your own home. Be certain to follow the directions *exactly*.

HYDROCOLLATOR PACKS

Equipment needed:
1. Hydrocollator pack, which is available from medical supply companies in the size desired. Instructions are printed on the box or will be found inside.
2. Large metal pan.
3. Terry covers which can be purchased with packs or thick terry towels which can be folded to provide six layers between the skin surface and the pack.

Technique:
1. Soak pack in cold water until it expands.
2. Immerse in pan of hot water.

3. Heat in hot water between 160°-175° for 15-20 minutes.
4. Remove pack and wrap in terry cover.
5. Apply pack to painful area for 20 minutes. Be certain there is adequate padding between the skin and pack.

Caution:
1. Additional layers of toweling may be added between skin and pack if the pack is too hot. Towels may be removed gradually as pack cools.
2. Keep pack in plastic bag in refrigerator when not in pan of water or in use.
3. A moist pack can be frozen to use as a cold pack if desired. Be certain to use enough padding between skin and pack.

HOT PARAFFIN BATH

Equipment needed:
1. Large (3 quart) double boiler.
2. ⅓ cup of mineral oil to each pound of paraffin.
3. 3-4 pounds of paraffin.
4. Candy thermometer.
5. Paper bags or towels for wrapping.
6. Rubber bands.

Technique:
1. Wash and dry hands. Remove all jewelry.
2. Place mineral oil and paraffin in top of double boiler with adequate water in bottom section. Heat slowly

37

and carefully over low heat to 126°F. Remove from heat. If a thermometer is not available, heat just till melted. Remove from heat and place on padded surface away from flame or burner, as paraffin is highly flammable. Allow wax to cool until a thin coating of white wax forms on the top.

3. Hold hands in a steady position with fingers slightly separated. Dip your hands alternately into and out of the wax, working quickly. Re-dip 10-15 times, allowing wax to cool on hands slightly between dippings. Do *not* move wrist or fingers once dipping is begun. This would cause a crack and the liquid wax could seep inside the "glove" and cause a burn.
4. Wrap the coated part in a paper bag and fasten around the wrist with a rubber band, or wrap old towels around the entire hand. Leave wrapped for 20 minutes.
5. Unwrap and peel off wax, which may be returned to the pan and be used again.

Caution:

1. Be extremely cautious in using wax because it is highly flammable.
2. Have another person present to help if possible.
3. Do not use if you have open cuts or other wounds on hands.
4. Wax may be applied to larger areas by using a paint brush to apply a layer at a time. Be careful not to drip wax where it may flare up.

HOT AND COLD CONTRAST

Definition: This alternate hot and cold application is used to relieve pain and congestion. It is particularly effective in reducing swelling. It can be done by immersing arms or legs in tubs, pails, or pans of water or can be applied to the body with packs.

Temperature:

Hot: 105°-110°
Cold: 60°-65°

Technique:

1. Contrast to arms or legs
   a. Prepare hot tub and cold tub.
   b. Start with hot tub for 3 minutes.
   c. Alternate to cold tub for 1 minute.
   d. Continue alternating between hot and cold tubs for 20-30 minutes.
   e. Always end with cold.

2. Contrast to body areas
   a. Prepare hot and cold packs.
   b. Place towel layers between the body part and pack.
   c. Place hot pack on body part for 3 minutes.

39

d. Place cold pack on body part for 1 minute.
e. Alternate cold and hot packs for 20-30 minutes.
f. Always end with cold.

CHAPTER FOUR

Gait and Functional Skills

The more chronic and long-standing the arthritic conditions, the more likely it is that difficulties in physical function will arise. The stresses and strains placed upon painful joints begin to show up in the form of difficulties when standing, walking, climbing stairs, and performing the functional activities necessary for daily living. In the patient with arthritis, the tolerance for activity diminishes, and fatigue may also reduce overall functional capacity. Since the basic aim of treatment in arthritis is to maintain and to restore maximum independence, this chapter will focus upon gait and ambulation and a limited area of functional problems.

When we speak of function, we are talking about the special, normal, or proper action of any part. If normal function is impaired, an assessment of the weaknesses and determination of realistic goals must be made prior to prescribing treatment. The functional goals for patients will vary with age, sex, occupation, and other factors. For example, the older retired patient may adjust more easily to lesser capability than the younger patient whose whole life demands higher performance goals.

The special skills of the physical and occupational therapist are invaluable in determining the deficits in performance, in the setting of goals, and in helping the patient achieve these goals. The *physical* therapist will explain techniques for relief of pain and help the patient with exercises to improve range of motion and to increase muscle strength and stability. She can help with gait training and suggest any adaptive devices needed. The *occupational* therapist will assist in splinting and bracing and be primarily concerned with self-care and daily living activities.

Since both the physical and occupational therapist are interested in the maximum independence of the patient, their roles frequently overlap. Both must exercise care in providing properly fitted and effectively designed devices which the patient can accept and use advantageously. They should not overburden the patient with a lot of worthless gadgets he does not need or will not use. Nor should they encourage the patient in the premature use of helping devices which promote dependency and which he does not yet need.

The weight-bearing joints in the hip, knee, ankle, and foot are subject to great stress in ambulation. We will discuss very generally the anatomy, deformities, and the methods of correction as they pertain to each of these individual joints. Let's start with the foot and proceed upward to the hip.

THE FOOT

Anatomically, there are two areas of major involvement in the foot: the subtalar joint and the metatarsophalangeal joints. (See Figure 9a.) Destruction of the joint surfaces and the ligaments supporting the small subtalar joint results in a gradual lateral deviation of the foot; this is referred to as a valgus deformity. (See Figure 9b.) Weight

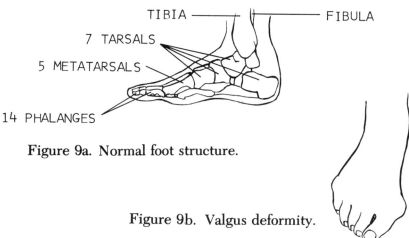

TIBIA ———— FIBULA

7 TARSALS

5 METATARSALS

14 PHALANGES

Figure 9a. Normal foot structure.

Figure 9b. Valgus deformity.

of the body then shifts to the inside border of the foot and places abnormal pressure on the first metatarsal joint. The medial and lateral plantar nerves may be compressed, producing pain and symptoms of tarsal tunnel syndrome. When the first metatarsal bone deviates medially, or turns in, the great toe will turn outward or laterally. This toe is of particular importance since it alone performs the final push-off in walking, and deformity and pain from bunions can render it ineffective. Misalignments and dislocations of many or all of the joints of the lesser toes produce the claw-toe deformity and resultant painful calluses. Painful feet frequently cause a limp, poor standing posture, and poor balance.

The best way to prevent and correct foot problems is to avoid "shoes in fashion" and select a properly fitted, well-constructed shoe which affords good support for balance and walking. The last of the shoe should be determined by the shape of the foot; the heel should fit snugly and the width at the ball must be adequate to prevent the squeezing of the toes together. In most cases it is not necessary to have special shoes made since shoe stores offer a wide variety of styles. Should you or your doctor feel that you need corrective devices, it is important that you select shoes which can accommodate such devices. These therapeutic corrections are made in the shoe itself or added to the sole and heel. They consist of pads, bars, and wedges. The purpose of these orthopedic supports is to relieve pressure by redistribution of weight, and to promote better walking patterns and posture. Appropriate exercise of the foot and ankle musculature may help to maintain joint stability. If these conservative measures fail, reconstructive foot surgery may be recommended to relieve pain and maintain function.

THE KNEE

The knee is a large, complex gliding joint which not only bends and straightens, but also has a slight ability to rotate. The large thigh or quadriceps muscles, assisted by several ligaments, provide the major stabilizing force of the knee joint. In degenerative arthritis, changes due to inflammation of the synovial lining, previous injury, and/ or abnormal stress produce wear on the joint surfaces, which become thinned and eroded. Calcification and loss of joint space cause instability and allow the knee to move abnormally. Secondarily, the quadriceps muscles become weak from disuse; contractures and spur formations develop and there is overall joint dysfunction. With continued deterioration there is most often flexure contraction, or inability to straighten the knee, constant pain, and changes in alignment which result in knock knee or bow leg deformity.

Conservative treatment varies; injections of corticosteriods, physical therapy modalities, muscle strengthening exercises, and restrictions of weight-bearing activities such as stair climbing may be recommended. At times it may be necessary to use a cane, crutches, or a walker to lessen the weight and the stress on the knee joint. Some protection can be given by the use of knee supports, splints, and braces. Often, a simple shoe correction may prove helpful. When these conservative measures fail, reconstructive surgery using the appropriate procedure—synovectomy, osteotomy, or arthroplasty, with or without prostheses—may be indicated.

THE HIP

Anatomically, the hip joint is designed to permit motion in six directions: flexion, extension, abduction, adduction, and internal and external rotation. Four major muscle groups provide stability and power. They are

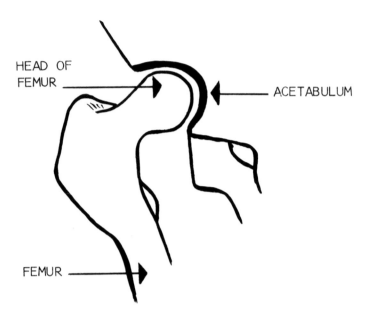

Figure 10. "Ball and socket" joint.

assisted by a strong capsule and ligaments. This versatile joint is referred to as a "ball and socket" since the top of the femur fits into the hip socket, which is called the acetabulum. In standing, there is equal pressure on both femoral heads; however, when one foot is lifted in walking, the force on the opposite hip is increased to three times the body weight.

Too often, hip problems are not diagnosed until late, when X-ray changes are already apparent and irreversible. In patients with traumatic and degenerative arthritis as well as those with rheumatoid arthritis, the predominant complaint is pain. As pain continues, motion becomes restricted, muscles become weak, and ambulation is difficult. As the degenerative process of the hip joint progresses, the bone becomes malaligned and impacted or jammed into the hip socket. This deformity essentially shortens the affected leg, sometimes as much as two or three inches. A limp then develops as a result of the leg length difference, muscle weakness, and pain. Because limping requires a greater expenditure of energy than do normal gait patterns, correction of the limp is vital if the patient is to continue to perform activity without fatiguing rapidly. A limp may be corrected by a built-up shoe and/or by using a cane, crutches, or a walker to relieve pressure and weight. Should the usual conservative treatment as described for the knee fail, there are a number of reconstructive procedures now available. Surgical procedures such as arthrodesis (or hip fusion), cup arthroplasty, correction of osteonecrosis of the femoral head, and total hip replacement often require a long period of immobilization and rehabilitation but have met with good success in relieving symptoms of arthritis of the hip joint.

The patient with marked hip and knee joint involvement has other significant problems in addition to limitations in walking and climbing stairs. He may find that getting into bed, using the toilet or bathtub, and driving or riding in a car are difficult, if not impossible. Blocks used to raise the furniture to a convenient height for sitting and standing and foot boards with attached pull-up devices to assist movements in bed help reduce patient effort and stress on joints. Common adaptations such as grab rails adjacent to the bathtub, shower, or toilet permit the patient to push or pull himself into position with safety. Elevated toilet seats and various styles of stools and chairs to use in the tub and shower are available.

In discussing the joints of the leg, it is easy to understand how each joint is interdependent upon the others in all modes of ambulation. One other very important area of consideration is the spine, because involvement of any segment of the cervical, thoracic, or lumbar vertebrae can present special postural problems. At least 40 percent of all orthopedic practice is related to this region. It is easy to appreciate that there is a vast range of disorders which can affect this intricate system of mobile joints. When there is pain in any area of the back, or a structural derangement causes a departure from the normal spinal alignment, there is usually some accompanying functional deficit.

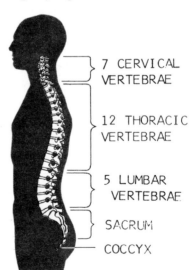

7 CERVICAL VERTEBRAE

12 THORACIC VERTEBRAE

5 LUMBAR VERTEBRAE

SACRUM

COCCYX

Figure 11. The spine.

A marked protrusion of the neck or a wry neck may indicate the presence of partial dislocation of cervical vertebrae and arthritis. With this condition there is restricted motion, which may be accompanied by pain radiating down the arm, pain at the back of the head, and muscle spasm and weakness. Instructing the patient in avoidance of neck stress is essential and requires an analysis of work, rest, and sleep habits. Sudden movement of the neck backward and into rotation as in driving a car must be avoided. Adjustments of seat and/or desk height at work or changes of posture in activities such as reading, writing, TV viewing, and sewing may be necessary. Certain athletic pursuits or habitual sleep postures may provoke symptoms, so these should be evaluated. Over 70 percent of the patients are helped by cervical traction, which can be done at home by using the Sayre

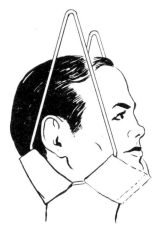

Figure 12. Sayre head halter.

49

head halter. Another valuable aid is the cervical collar. During ambulatory activities, the collar helps to restrain motion and reduce nerve pressure. The collar may be made of soft foam rubber, firm felt, or hard plastic. An elastic chin strap or cervical pillow may be used while sleeping.

Symptoms of pain, limited function, and excessive fatiguability should not be ignored by the arthritic whose less flexible back is more vulnerable to stress. These warning signs can alert you to a more frequent and careful inspection of your postural and gait habits. Stooped shoulders or a hunched back show that the normal curve in the back is increased, and a condition of the upper back known as kyphosis may develop. When the low back curve is exaggerated in a swayback position, it is known as lordosis. Still another spinal deviation is scoliosis, which

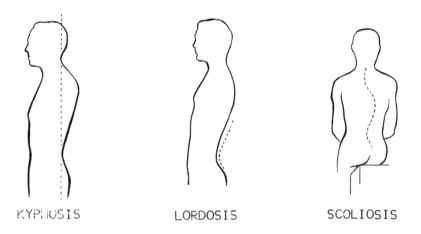

KYPHOSIS   LORDOSIS   SCOLIOSIS

Figure 13.

50

may be either a C- or S-shaped lateral curvature of the spine.

Any of these conditions, if allowed to progress, can cause changes in the bones, muscular spasm and weakness, and functional changes in the vital organs. Some rules to follow in order to avoid wear and tear on the spine are: 1) substitute squatting for bending over from the waist, 2) avoid heavy lifting and pushing and pulling of heavy objects, and 3) use a cart with wheels or other labor-saving devices to move or carry heavy objects. Back supports and braces may be prescribed because they restrict the wearer from performing activities which increase back pain. The single, reliably effective back support has not been devised, which is probably the reason that they often lie unused in the closet.

Functional testing, which determines weaknesses, helps the physician to anticipate the problems and assess the need for self-help aids. In the case of leg weaknesses, it may be necessary to prescribe the use of some aid to share the weight when walking. The decision to use a wheelchair, glider chair, crutches, walker, or cane can be made after considering the patient's total health condition and his work and home environment. An important fact, which the patient frequently cannot accept, is that the use of a crutch or cane does not mean he is going downhill or becoming a cripple. Often it is a temporary and preventive measure to protect a joint from becoming permanently damaged and deformed. For the already handicapped individual, it can be a permanent means of ambulation.

The cane is usually the aid of choice when only minimal weight relief or balance correction is needed. The cane is usually held in the hand on the same side as the involved leg. It is moved forward with that leg in order to absorb a part of the body weight. Measuring for the correct length of the cane can be done while standing erect with the cane held slightly forward and to the side of the foot. Proper height allows the elbow to be bent about 30°. If an adjustable cane is not used, the standard 36″ cane can be cut to the desired length and a good rubber suction tip placed on the end for safety. The conventional "C" shaped handle may be substituted for a "T" or functional handle when hand limitations are present.

If crutches are recommended, they must be correctly fitted and carefully selected according to type and style, and the patient must receive supervised instructions and practice in using them skillfully and safely. A variety of crutch styles and specialized adaptations are available. The type selected will be determined by the patient's limitations in strength and motion of the shoulder, arms, wrists, and hands. Relieving the stress from the legs should not be done at the risk of destroying the arms and hands. Any crutch or added supports should be constructed from lightweight materials. If crutches are too long, they may cause discomfort or injury to the shoulder; if too short, they encourage bad posture habits; if they are too heavy, the stress will be increased rather than decreased.

The most common type is the axillary or underarm crutch. Rubber foam cushions to prevent pressure should cover the shoulder piece and the hand grip. A good suction tip should be applied to the bottom ends for safety. In measuring, allow a one-inch (1″) space between shoulder pad and the armpit. The hand grip should be adjusted so that in the standing position there is about a thirty-degree (30°) bend at each elbow. As you apply pressure in walking, the elbow will almost straighten and the shoulder piece will be supported against the side of the chest. *Never* lean or "hang" on the shoulder piece in standing or walking.

The Canadian or Loftstrand crutch fits across the back of the arm to give added support in case of weakness of the triceps muscles. When the arms are severely involved, and especially when the standard hand grip exaggerates deformity of the hand, a forearm platform is recommended. This permits weight distribution over the entire forearm and protects the weakened joints of the wrist and hand.

How do you walk with crutches? The physical therapist should instruct the patient in the correct crutch technique for walking and stair management. Practice sessions should continue until the essential skills can be performed with confidence and safety. Maintaining good balance is usually easier if the feet are not placed too close together. Separate your feet to a distance which gives you the greatest stability. To avoid falls, take care when moving and placing the crutches on slick or heavily carpeted floors and on uneven or rough outdoor surfaces. Check for objects lying on the floor or ground and avoid throw rugs in particular. They are potentially dangerous and can do exactly that—throw you! Check the suction tips regularly for wear and for dirt build-up, which makes them ineffective.

The most elemental of crutch gaits is the four point gait. It is the slowest, but gives greatest stability and safety since there are always three points on the floor. Start with equal weight on both feet and both crutches. Move the right crutch forward. Move the left foot forward and shift your weight to the left foot and right crutch. Move the left crutch forward. Move the right foot forward and shift your weight to the right foot and left crutch. The two point gait is faster since there is a simultaneous movement of the crutch with the opposite leg. It resembles a normal walk, while allowing the crutch to share the load of the body weight. There are two points of support. The three point gait is used when one leg is more involved than the other. Both crutches and the weaker leg are moved forward at once and the stronger leg is brought forward to them.

When maneuvering stairs, it is important that the stronger leg lead when going up a step, with the weight supported on the crutches on the step below. The weaker leg and the crutches should lead when going down. If railings are available, they can be utilized with crutches as shown in Figure 14.

Some individuals find greater security in using a walker than in using a cane or crutches. Walkers are available in fixed or adjustable models, and can be fitted with carrying bags or trays and many convenience accessories. They should have rubber tips on the leg, not casters which move. You should always push down on a walker except when lifting it forward when walking. Place all four legs of the walker firmly on the floor for maximum safety when moving the walker forward.

A glider, which is a chair on wheels, is sometimes recommended to eliminate excessive walking and periods of standing. It is propelled by the feet and the hands are left free to perform household tasks or activities. It is smaller than a wheel chair, and so is more suitable when space is limited.

When arthritis becomes severely disabling, the wheel chair may be the solution. When selecting the chair which features the greatest comfort and help, you must consider that the patient will be transferring from the chair to bed, car, and toilet. It must be fitted properly to provide support where necessary and must permit the patient the mobility to continue home, vocational, and social functions. Many accessories such as lap boards can be added to the wheel chair, and ramps and other modifications can be added to the home to assist in independent living.

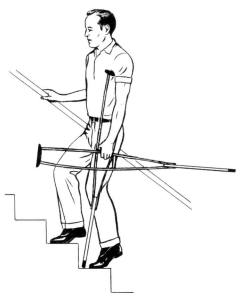

Figure 14. Using a railing with crutches.

Probably the greatest complaint of an arthritis patient with limited function is the inability to get out of the home. Travel and transport depend upon the availability of a car or a suitable public transportation system which accommodates the elderly or handicapped. The demands and suggestions made by you to your legislators at the national, state, and local level can help to improve public transportation.

In order to drive or ride in a car, the patient must, obviously, first be able to get in and out of the car. This skill has to be worked out on an individual basis after assessing the patient's physical limitations and the car itself. Generally speaking, it is easier to back up to the car seat, sit down, then pull the legs in. If turning the body and lifting the legs simultaneously is difficult, the use of a sliding seat cushion helps to rotate the buttocks on the seat of the car.

There are many aids to assist in opening the car door, key cases with built-up grips for turning on the ignition, spinner knobs for easier steering, and special arm rests for comfort. For the person with severely impaired functioning of the legs, the car can be modified to be completely operated by hand. Persons with limited neck range of motion can use a wide-angle mirror for increased visibility, and adjustable backrests add comfort on long trips.

CHAPTER FIVE

Self-Help Aids
and Daily Living

Energy conservation and joint protection are two very important concepts that anyone with arthritis should understand and attempt to put into practice in all the activities he does throughout each day. By following some suggestions we will give on energy conservation, much of the over-fatigue and excessive stress which can contribute to increased pain and further joint destruction can be avoided. Unbelievable as it may seem, the normal stress from picking up a book, taking a bath, or opening a door can lead to deformity. Yet, how can you eliminate these routine tasks which are essential for everyday living? Quite simply, you cannot. To remain functionally mobile and independent, each of us must perform activities of self-care, homemaking, and various other tasks required by our living patterns. Since you cannot eliminate these tasks, you must find easier ways to do them, and our time and energy savers can help you. By following the joint protection principles discussed here, you can avoid placing additional stress on weakened joints. It may be difficult to break long-established habits and routines. However, by carefully planning, pacing, and moderating activities, you can change the way you perform and still accomplish what you want and need to do.

We want to emphasize that not all of the material we will cover will apply to every person in every situation. Consideration of your personal life style and physical limitations should guide you in your decision to use any of the self-help devices we will discuss. You must continue to perform as many tasks as possible without using such devices; however, such aids should be used for joint protection during acute inflammatory stages and when joint deterioration has already restricted independent activity.

Several factors should be considered when selecting self-help aids. They should be simple and durable in design, lightweight, economical, versatile, pleasing to the eye, and, above all, useful. You must know why you are using the device and how to use it properly.

Although many different situational skills will be covered, we cannot encompass every area of daily living. Our suggestions may be used as guides when looking for appropriate aids and in using them, but you should also use your own judgment as to how practical and useful any particular item will be to you personally.

Before discussing specific situations, it is important to learn the basic principles of joint protection. These should always be utilized in all daily activities.

Self-Help Aids and Daily Living

1. Always use the strongest and/or largest joint possible to accomplish a task. Instead of using your fingers, use your wrist; instead of using your wrist, use your elbow; instead of using your elbow, use your shoulder. For example, use your palms to shut drawers, not your figertips or the side of your fingers.

2. Avoid excessive pressure against the backs of your fingers, the pads of your thumbs and fingers, and the thumb side of each finger. Pressures in these directions contribute to the dislocation of the large knuckle joints between the fingers and the palm, with subsequent ulnar deviation deformities of the fingers (Figure 15). Use your palms to help you rise from a chair, not your fingers. Do not prop your face on your fingers. When holding objects, hold them parallel to the knuckles, not diagonally across the palm. Pick up coffee cups and water glasses with both hands, keeping the fingers partially extended. Add lever-

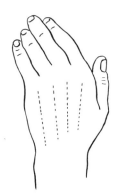

Figure 15.   Ulnar deviation.

age devices to faucets and doorknobs so that the palms, instead of the fingers, can be used to apply the necessary force.

3. *Avoid prolonged periods in the same position.* This includes everything from holding books, cards, or an iron to sitting or standing for a long period of time. Your position should be changed at least every half-hour when your large joints are involved, as in sitting or standing, and every few minutes if the small joints are involved. If you must maintain a tight grasp, the joints should be released often and completely relaxed. Avoid carrying handbags, shopping bags, pails, and baskets by the handles for long periods of time.

4. *Emphasize joint extension in all activities.* It is common for people with arthritis to develop flexure contractures such as shown in Figure 16. A slightly flexed joint position is more comfortable during periods of inflammation and pain, and most of our daily activities require positions where joints are flexed or bent. These positions must be counteracted with as much joint extension as possible. You should also remember that the extended position places less strain on the joints. For example, dust furniture with an open hand with the fingers extended, rather than by gripping the dustcloth with bent fingers and cupped hand.

5. *Avoid lifting whenever possible.* Try to slide heavy objects along a counter, or if they need to be transported to another room, put them on a cart with wheels. If you absolutely must lift something, use both hands with the palms facing upward and the weight of the object distributed to the larger wrist, elbow, and shoulder joints as

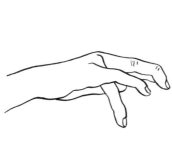

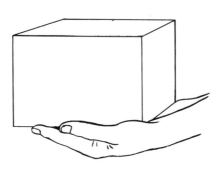

Figure 16. Flexure-contraction.

Figure 17. Proper lifting technique, using both hands with fingers extended.

shown in Figure 17. When lifting objects from the floor, always bend at the knees rather than the back. Use your entire body to open and close heavy doors and drawers.

6. *Place items conveniently so that you can work in a relaxed position to eliminate strain.* If the task will take more than ten minutes to complete, sit on a high kitchen stool with a good supportive back and a swivel seat.

Apply these principles as you evaluate your daily performance: 1) reduce the force, 2) change the method, 3) use energy-saving and joint protection equipment, 4) eliminate unnecessary activity, and 5) take intermittent rest periods. Remember these principles as we offer alternative methods for accomplishing some daily activities and discuss use of some of the more common self-help aids.

BATHING AND GROOMING

Because of the personal and private nature of bathing, toileting, grooming, and dressing activities, it is easy to understand the arthritic's desire to perform independently. After all, good grooming is very important to our morale and these are things that we feel we must do for ourselves.

Safety and convenience are prime considerations for the bathroom. Non-skid bathmats and skid-resistant strips placed in the tub or shower can protect you from falls. Grab bars or safety rails which have been installed strategically near the tub, shower, or toilet are good safety features and are helpful in getting up or down.

Self-Help Aids and Daily Living

Taking a bath can be a problem if you have hip and knee involvement. To reduce the strain when getting in and out of the tub, use a commercially available non-skid bath stool or chair or a bath seat board. Although you won't get down as low in the tub, you will be able to get out much easier. A shower caddy or a tub tray can keep bathing essentials close at hand. A bath mitt may be more convenient than a cloth for washing since it allows you to keep your fingers in the extended position. Long handled brushes extend limited reach and a shower hose can be helpful for rinsing. When drying your back, avoid a tight grasp on the towel by sewing loops at each end of it, then slip your elbows through to hold the towel, and let your shoulders do the drying. Or, simply put on a loose-fitting terrycloth robe and pat yourself dry.

Elevating the toilet seat four or more inches greatly reduces stress on the hips and knees. Raised toilet seats are available in many models and heights, some cushioned and even sporting arm rests!

The major difficulty in personal grooming is the inability to grip the small handles of the tooth brush, hair brush, comb, razor, and other small items. Since grasping tightly with weakened joints can be both painful and damaging, increasing the diameter of the handle by using cylindrical foam padding permits the fingers to relax. Limited reach caused by shoulder or elbow involvement can be overcome by lengthening the handle with an extension device. There are also commercial items on the market designed specifically for each of these tasks. Electric appliances such as tooth brushes, razors, hair brushes, dryers, and nail care items can also reduce manual energy expenditure.

Self-Help Aids and Daily Living

When you squeeze the tube of toothpaste, use the little finger side of your hand so that pressure on the finger pads and in the direction of ulnar deviation is avoided. Figure 18 shows the proper technique.

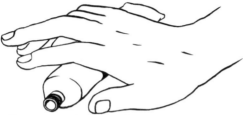

Figure 18. Proper technique for squeezing toothpaste tube.

If you keep your hair in a short, natural style it will be easier to wash and manage. If you set your hair, a Velcro type of roller can be easily managed with one hand. It has tiny hooks which grab the hair and does not require the use of pins or clips to hold it in place. Around-the-neck or wall extension mirrors allow hand-free viewing.

DRESSING

There are two main areas to be considered when discussing dressing. First, we must overcome the difficulties of limited reach, grasp, and bending. Next, we must select clothing which is easy to manage and care for, yet attractive. Loose-fitting clothing with front openings is easier to manage than pullovers or tight dresses or pants with back fasteners. A zipper pull such as the one in Figure 19a and zippers with big ring pulls can make dressing easier to manage. Buttons may also be a problem. You

64

Self-Help Aids and Daily Living

may want to use a button hook like the one shown in Figure 19b or replace the buttons with Velcro fasteners, which are available at most sewing stores. Velcro makes an ideal fastener for hard-to-manage places such as shirt collars, undergarments, and for outer garments.

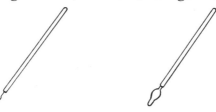

Figure 19a. Button hook.   Figure 19b. Zipper pull.

If it is impossible to reach your feet, use a long-handled shoe horn to put on shoes. When hand involvement prevents you from tying, replace the standard shoe laces with elastic ones or have a zipper inserted which can be opened and closed with a zipper pull. Buckle-type straps may be replaced by Velcro closures. A lowered closet rod and convenient shelves and drawers will also help simplify the dressing process.

HOMEMAKING

Architectural barriers could be eliminated if we all had the opportunity to build a "dream house." Since this is usually out of the question, inexpensive adaptations and rearrangement of the existing furniture in your present home or apartment may be the answer to everyday functional problems. We will not go into the many modifications necessitated by wheelchair living, such as

65

entry ways, stairs, wider doors, and so forth. Publications from the federal Department of Health, Education and Welfare and from other organizations concerned with architectural barriers to the handicapped can be consulted for extensive remodeling if necessary. Since you may be sitting down more than the average person does, chairs, sofas, and tables should be selected carefully. A well-designed chair provides good body support, gives you adequate leverage to regain a standing position, offers arm rests, and should be comfortable and adaptable to your needs. Tables should be sturdy, the correct height as correlated to the seat of the chair, and should provide adequate work space.

When you have analyzed and made your home more functional, the next step is maintaining it. When you have arthritis, any activity requires more effort and energy than it normally would, and so it is important to plan your work ahead. Conserve your energy by spacing work periods throughout the day and allowing for regular rest periods. Rest *before* you feel tired, and try not to begin a complicated activity when you are not up to it or know it will take longer than your endurance will allow. If there are any chores which cause undue strain, consider letting another family member or friend do them. It is up to you to protect your joints by evaluating which tasks cause prolonged pain, then finding alternative methods of accomplishing the task or letting someone else do it for you.

To make the bed, straighten your fingers when smoothing the sheets. Save steps by working only once around the bed, completing each corner before going on to the

Self-Help Aids and Daily Living

next, and tucking all the bedclothes in at one time. You can protect painful fingers by tucking bedclothes in with a wooden paddle or using elasticized fitted sheets. Select lightweight and easy-to-care-for bedding.

It is a good idea to keep cleaning supplies in various rooms of the house in order to avoid unnecessary steps and to conserve energy. Items can be transported from room to room by using a cart with wheels, a dolly with casters, or by wearing an apron with large pockets to carry a number of small items. Select lightweight cleaning implements which require little or no lifting and which can be used while practicing good body mechanics. Keep this in mind when choosing vacuum cleaners and mops. Both are difficult to use, and you must investigate the features of each unit before deciding which is best for you.

When cleaning, use a sponge rather than a cloth or paper towel, because you will find it easier to squeeze the water out by pushing down on the sponge with your palm than it is to wring out a cloth. A long-handled sponge can assist in cleaning the bathtub, and a shower hose can be used to rinse it afterwards. If you use a liquid cleaner to clean windows and mirrors, push the plunger down with the palm of your hand and keep your fingers extended when wiping.

Also keep your fingers extended when dusting. The use of a dust mitt will make this easier and can even make dusting a helpful exercise. Remember to use a counter-clockwise motion if you are right-handed, or clockwise if you are left-handed. One other item which you may find useful when cleaning is a long-handled dustpan to eliminate fatigue and strain from unnecessary bending.

Self-Help Aids and Daily Living

Automatic washers and dryers and the excellent new washing products and fabrics which cut down on hand scrubbing and ironing time have certainly transformed "wash-day" since the days of the wooden wash tub and galvanized scrub board! A few additional hints to lighten laundry tasks are to use a laundry cart, to keep cleaning products close to where they are used, and to use a long-handled reacher to load and unload clothing. You must remember not to pick up objects such as large boxes and jugs of bleach and laundry powder. Some reachers have magnets attached to them which permit picking up pins, paper clips, and other tiny metal objects which are difficult to pick up when grasp and bending are restricted.

If you must do hand washing, never wring out clothes with a twisting motion. Figure 20 shows how to reduce

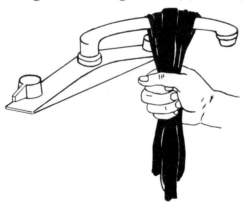

Figure 20. Proper technique for wringing clothes.

the stress on the wrist and finger joints. You can also wrap the clothes around the water faucet and squeeze or pull to remove the water. If you hang clothes on the line, use the

68

push-on rather than the spring-type clothes pins. Conserve energy while you sort or fold laundry or iron by sitting on a stool. Ironing boards are available which have a height adjustment. Maintain a loose grasp on the iron, using either large circular motions in a counter-clockwise direction or long sweeping strokes in order to maintain or increase shoulder and elbow motion. Travel irons are much lighter than regular ones and may be easier to use. However, if you choose clothes wisely, buying knits or the permanent press type when possible, you may be able to eliminate all or most of your ironing.

KITCHEN PLANNING/MEAL PREPARATION

For many homemakers, meal preparation is the most physically demanding of all household tasks. We spend considerable time in the kitchen, but most kitchens are poorly designed for the person with marked physical limitations. When the sink and counter top are unreachable and appliances cannot be managed without help, major remodelling may be necessary. However, less expensive and drastic measures can help to overcome some of the barriers. Consider reducing food preparation time and work by taking advantage of convenience foods such as frozen vegetables, cake mixes, and other easy-to-prepare products. Sit rather than stand for long periods in order to conserve energy. A high stool with a swivel seat can help you to reach the sink or stove. Rearrange work areas and reorganize storage areas so as to avoid excessive bending and lifting. Heavy utensils should be kept on the counter or as close to waist height as possible. A pegboard in an easy-to-reach area provides a simple yet decorative method of storage for pots and pans. Dividers in drawers or lazy susans help to make utensils more accessible.

When purchasing kitchen items, consider the weight of the object; cast iron pans are not for you! The lighter the better, so try to use plastic, stainless steel, or aluminum dishes and mixing bowls, and aluminum, stainless steel, or lightweight porcelain pots and pans. Electric can openers, knives, mixers, and blenders help prevent strain on your hands and conserve your energy. If you do not have an electric can opener, at least try to get the swing-away type which screws on the wall. The regular hand crank can opener should not be used if you have weakened, painful hands. If you don't have an electric

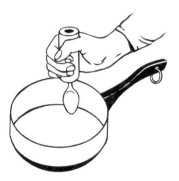

Figure 21. Correct way to stir with spoon.

mixer and must do your mixing by hand, hold the spoon with a cylinder grasp and turn in a counter-clockwise direction with the right hand. This position helps to maintain the wrist and fingers in a straight position. Also, do not hold the mixing bowl too tightly. There are several methods which can be used to help to stabilize the bowl: 1) Place a wet cloth under the bowl, 2) use a wooden bowl holder or 3) use a commercially available bowl such as a stainless steel one with a stand or the type with a large bottom suction cup. The stand for the stainless steel bowl also allows you to turn the bowl on its side in order to pour or scrape out the contents. An alternative method would be to place a wet cloth over an empty pot and put a slightly smaller bowl inside the pot over the cloth at an angle. The traction from the cloth holds the bowl in place, thus taking strain from the one hand which would have had to support the entire weight of the bowl.

To prepare vegetables, use a vegetable peeler which allows you to slip all your fingers into it or use with the fingers extended. Use a four-sided grater rather than the flat type, and stabilize it with the palm of your hand on top. A cutting board with two aluminum nails helps to hold vegetables in place while you chop or peel.

When opening jars, you can prevent ulnar deviation by opening them with the right hand and closing them with the left hand. One method of opening a jar is to place it on a rubber mat to prevent slipping, then press down with the heel of the hand and turn. There are several jar openers which fasten underneath the cupboard, and the V-shaped type which attaches to the wall is widely available also. Do not close jars too tightly; you want to use less force to reopen them.

A pan holder is useful in keeping the pan in place on the burner. This device attaches to the stove with suction cups and clamps onto the handle. It keeps the pan from

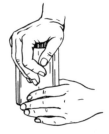

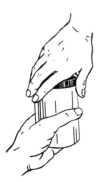

Figure 22a. Correct way to open jar.

Figure 22b. Incorrect way to open jar.

turning and frees your hand. Never try to lift a heavy pot; instead, slide it along the counter top to the sink if possible. The contents can then be easily removed if you use a frying insert or a special spaghetti cooker, also known as a food blancher, which has a perforated insert fitted neatly inside. When removing something from the oven, use an oven shovel or mitt-type potholder and lift the pan with both palms. Once everything is ready to be served, place it all on a cart with wheels in order to avoid the strain of carrying and making countless trips back and forth.

After preparing the meal, be sure to soak your dirty pots and pans in order to make cleaning up easier. If you wash your dishes by hand, sit on a stool. The stool is the proper height if you are able to touch the bottom of the sink easily with the palms of your hands. A simple wash mitt is perfect for keeping your fingers in extension while you scrub; remember to use a counter-clockwise motion if you're right-handed, and a clockwise motion if you are left-handed.

Eating. Standard eating utensils may require modifications such as the following:

1. When grasp is limited or weak, handles of forks, knives, and spoons can be built up with foam padding or a bicycle handle grip. If grasp is totally lacking, you can use an elastic band which goes around the hand and has a pocket to hold the utensil.

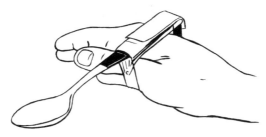

Figure 23. Utensil holder.

2. A long-handled extendor can help you reach for objects.

3. When there is restricted motion of the forearm with the palm facing up, called supination, a swivel spoon can help compensate for the lack of motion.

A plate guard which consists of a detachable metal or plastic rim gives a surface to push food against, and a suction cup on the bottom of the plate prevents its sliding. Handles on cups which are large or shaped like a T are easier to pick up. Jackets of stretch terry cloth on glasses or flexible straws may aid in drinking.

MISCELLANEOUS

A quad phone grip can be attached to the receiver of the phone. You can slip your whole hand in to hold the phone, and exercise your fingers while you talk!

A doorknob attachment adds leverage to the handle, thus allowing you to use the palm of your hand rather than your fingers to open the door. It may help to add some

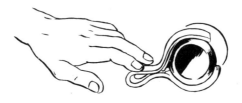

Figure 24.   Doorknob extender.

leverage to keys, faucets, lamp switches, and other small knobs and items which must be rotated. Some devices designed specifically for these purposes are available through mail order houses and some retail outlets such as drug stores.

Many different types of writing aids are available which prevent the static positioning required to hold a pencil. When writing, you can increase the circumference of the pencil by using foam padding or sticking the pencil through a small rubber ball. The utensil holder which wraps around the palm and is used for holding eating utensils can also hold a pencil. Typing is actually preferable to writing and is easier if you have an electric typewriter. Manual scissors are especially hard on the joints, so if you have electric scissors, use them.

When reading, use a book rest or prop the book up on some pillows; if you play cards, use a card holder to avoid keeping your fingers constantly in the same position.

We have tried to choose common situations which are encountered in daily living and suggest practical modifications and solutions. If you are able to function without using self-help aids you are fortunate, and we urge you to continue doing so. Remember that the use of gadgets can be self-defeating if they are used prematurely and if they cause you to avoid the exercise you need.

On the following pages, the principles of joint protection have been summarized for your convenience in referring to them. Hints on saving time and energy also are listed.

TIME AND ENERGY SAVERS

1. Plan activities in advance and with moderation in order to avoid excessive physical and emotional stress and over-fatigue.

2. Organize and re-arrange rooms and work areas for efficiency and convenience. For example, in the kitchen, store or place objects you will use together in convenient locations so that you don't have to waste steps collecting them every time you need to use them.

3. Plan an easy flow of work; an assembly line accomplishes more with less time and effort. For example, take *all* vegetables or other food for the meal to the sink, prepare them, take them to the stove and cook them, then serve them. This saves many trips from refrigerator to sink to stove to table.

4. Use wheels to transport instead of carrying. Use large pockets or bags to carry several small items. For example, put all food on a wheeled cart and take it to the table, then collect all left-overs and dishes on the cart and return them to the kitchen.

5. Adjust work heights to eliminate excessive bending, reaching, and straining in all activities.

6. Sit rather than stand. For example, use a stool when ironing.

7. Use gravity to assist you. For example, a laundry chute can save steps into the cellar.

8. Provide a quiet, well-lighted, and well-ventilated atmosphere.

9. Use modern labor-saving devices, lightweight utensils, easy-to-care-for clothing, and other devices to avoid unnecessary work.

10. Alternate periods of activity with rest periods. A lying position uses ⅓ less energy than standing. For example, plan ten minutes of rest for each hour of activity.

Self-Help Aids and Daily Living

PRINCIPLES OF JOINT PROTECTION

1. Always use the strongest and/or largest joint possible to accomplish a task.

   Instead of using your fingers, use your wrist; instead of using your wrist, use your elbow; and instead of using your elbow, use your shoulder.

2. Avoid excessive pressure against the backs of your fingers, the pads of your thumbs and fingers, and the lateral (or thumb) side of each finger.

   Dislocation of joints and muscle imbalance can be caused by pressures in these directions. Avoid this by using proper positioning when holding onto objects and adding leverage devices to faucets, doorknobs, and keys. Hold with object parallel to knuckles, not across the palm diagonally.

3. Avoid prolonged periods of holding in the same position.

   Change your position frequently: Try to do so every half hour when sitting or standing and every few minutes when holding things with your hands. Especially avoid using a tight grip.

4. Emphasize joint extension in all activities.

   This position places less strain on your joints and counteracts the tendency toward flexion (bent) deformities.

5. Avoid lifting whenever possible.

   Use alternative, less stress-producing methods to move objects. If you must lift, use both hands with the palms facing upward to distribute the weight to the larger joints.

6. Place items conveniently so you can work in a relaxed position with strain eliminated.

Apply these principles to your performance in any of the following ways by: (1) reducing the force, (2) changing the method, (3) using energy saving and joint protecting equipment, (4) eliminating the activity, and (5) taking intermittent rest periods.

CHAPTER SIX

Medications in Arthritis

The treatment of an arthritic condition may include any or all of the modalities available today. Medication is the most common form of treatment prescribed by physicians, but physical therapy, rest (either of the whole body or a part), and surgery are the other potential approaches. This multidisciplinary concept should be kept in mind while we are discussing the drug treatment of arthritis.

Ultimately, any drug program is aimed at the relief of pain. Pain, in turn, is due to inflammation in the joints and, at times, in the surrounding tissues. If pain is relieved, then the accompanying stiffness and swelling will have an opportunity to improve. The medications discussed here will be primarily anti-inflammatory drugs.

The selection of the appropriate medicine or medicines for any individual patient is a complicated task for the physician. Each of the almost 100 forms of arthritis has its own drug or group of drugs which may be of value. Many of these drugs are useful in more than one type of arthritis. In many cases, a combination of drugs is needed in treating the patient. It is a process of trial and error with most patients in order to find the most effective therapeutic program. The following medications are used in arthritis treatment:

SALICYLATES

The salicylates are a group of chemicals, the most common of which is aspirin. Aspirin is sold under many brand names, often in combination with other drugs, such as in Excedrin and Anacin. Aspirin itself may be modified chemically to form a compound which contains sodium (sodium salicylate) or magnesium (Mobidin). These combinations may be less irritating to the stomach. A liquid preparation, choline salicylate, is sold as Arthropan. It also may be somewhat less irritating to the stomach than aspirin. Regardless of the chemical make-up or associated drugs in the preparation, a salicylate is the anti-inflammatory drug in these compounds.

It should be emphasized that salicylates are anti-inflammatory in arthritis, not just analgesic. That is, instead of being painkillers only, aspirin-type drugs actually work against inflammation. Unfortunately, the analgesic effect of aspirin is much more widely appreciated than its anti-inflammatory capability. This, plus the fact that aspirin is sold without prescription, tends to lessen its reputation among patients and physicians alike.

Aspirin and its sister compounds are potentially useful in all forms of arthritis except acute gout. In rheumatoid arthritis, aspirin alone will give substantial relief to 50 percent of patients. In order that a patient obtain a good effect from aspirin, however, it must be used in substantial doses. Ten to fifteen aspirin tablets per day should be used before its effectiveness can be judged. Although many patients are concerned with taking this number of tablets of aspirin per day, most will tolerate it quite well. Some arthritis patients will notice side effects such as abdominal pain or ringing of the ears at these dose levels. Adjusting the dosage under medical direction usually relieves these side effects. Before using aspirin for arthritis, the patient should consult with his physician, because aspirin should not be used simultaneously with certain prescription drugs.

INDOCIN (INDOMETHACIN)

Indocin is a quite widely used anti-inflammatory drug. It is potentially useful in all types of arthritis, but much more effective in some types, such as gout, than in others, such as rheumatoid arthritis. It is also effective in osteoarthritis, particularly of the hip and knee. Initial enthusiasm for this drug has dampened over the years, but it does have some beneficial effect in most arthritis cases. Like most arthritis medications, Indocin may cause stomach upset. It may also cause dizziness and intense headache.

BUTAZOLIDIN-TYPE DRUGS

Butazolidin is the leading member of a group of drugs which are all quite similar. Butazolidin is most commonly marketed as Butazolidin-Alka, which is Butazolidin plus antacid; it is also made under another brand name as

Azolid. Tandearil, a sister compound, is also sold as Oxalid. Butazolidin, Butazolidin-Alka, Azolid, Tandearil, and Oxalid all have essentially the same capability in the treatment of arthritis. They are excellent in the treatment of acute gout attacks, tendonitis, and bursitis. They are less effective in rheumatoid arthritis and osteoarthritis. Because of their potentially toxic effect on bone marrow, these compounds must be used very cautiously in patients who receive them as long-term therapy. As with other arthritis medicines, this group of drugs commonly causes stomach upset. They may also cause rash, dizziness, and fluid retention.

ANTIMALARIAL DRUGS

It has been observed that drugs originally developed for treatment of malaria also are somewhat effective in rheumatoid arthritis and one of its sister diseases, lupus erythematosus. Plaquenil and Aralen are the antimalarial drugs most commonly used in these conditions. Although some physicians are enthusiastic about the use of these compounds, their potentially harmful effect on vision has discouraged widespread use.

GOLD

Gold shots have been used in the treatment of rheumatoid arthritis for many years. Much mystery and misinformation exists concerning both safety and effectiveness of gold treatment. Gold is extremely valuable in the early stages of rheumatoid arthritis. While most medications can only suppress or "cover" the disease, many arthritis specialists feel that gold may actually be curative in some patients with rheumatoid arthritis. Despite the enthusiasm for gold treatment by arthritis specialists, many physicians and patients are hesitant to undertake this mode of treatment. Two major misconceptions form the basis for this negative opinion: First, it has been said by some that gold is not effective therapy. This is due to poor selection of patients by the physicians. Remember, gold is valuable in rheumatoid arthritis and *only* rheumatoid arthritis. It is not effective in any other form of arthritis. Therefore, the patients with other types of arthritis such as osteoarthritis, gout, or other variant forms of rheumatoid arthritis are not benefited by gold therapy. Also contributing to the many gold treatment failures are those patients with rheumatoid arthritis who could benefit from gold treatment but who are not treated for an adequate period of time before the gold is stopped. Gold treatment, which is given by injection, is effective only after at least ten and perhaps up to twenty shots, but rarely before that. Discontinuation of treatment before this time contributes to many unjustified failures in gold therapy.

The second deterrent to gold treatment is the misconception that gold therapy is dangerous. To the contrary, this drug is perhaps one of the safest forms of treatment of rheumatoid arthritis. It must, however, be given under the supervision of doctors and nurses who are familiar with its potential side effects. The side effects include rash, nephritis (inflammation of the kidneys), and bone marrow changes.

Medications in Arthritis

TOLECTIN (TOLMETIN SODIUM)

Nearly 200 compounds have been developed by drug companies throughout the world recently. Four have been approved by the Food and Drug Administration of our federal government in the past two years. Tolectin is one of these new compounds which are currently available, but is a distant relative of Indocin. Unlike Indocin, Tolectin is relatively well tolerated by most patients. It is uniquely effective in some patients and of the same value as aspirin in other patients. It has been used successfully in most types of arthritis in tests performed in this and other countries.

Tolectin shares with the other new drugs a number of potential side effects including headache, dizziness, stomach upset, and diarrhea. It is somewhat less irritating to the stomach than the previously described drugs except for gold, which has no harmful effect on the stomach.

MOTRIN (IBUPROFEN), NALFON (FENOPROFEN CALCIUM), AND NAPROSYN (NAPROXEN)

These three drugs are all sister compounds. Motrin was the first of the group to be released for use in this country. The other two, Nalfon and Naprosyn, were placed on the market simultaneously with Tolectin in 1976. All three of these drugs are potentially useful in most types of arthritis. Each is uniquely effective on certain patients while being only moderately so in other patients. Although these drugs are similar enough to share the same potential side effects, each is dissimilar enough to be worth trying on a patient who has failed to respond to the sister compounds of the group.

Many arthritis specialists try Motrin, Nalfon, Naprosyn and Tolectin until one is found to be effective. The exact sequence in which they are used depends on the individual preference of the doctor.

Like Tolectin, these drugs may cause dizziness, headache, stomach upset, and diarrhea. Also, as with Tolectin, these compounds are less irritating than aspirin for most patients.

CORTISONE-TYPE DRUGS

When cortisone was first given to patients in 1950, it was heralded as the miracle cure for rheumatoid arthritis. Unbridled enthusiasm led to aggressive use of cortisone in all types of arthritis. The use of large doses of cortisone seemed to cause severe side effects in many patients. It was then recognized that cortisone and its derivatives are all double-edged swords in the fight to cure arthritis. This appreciation of the toxic effects of long-term cortisone usage has led to a more conservative approach to its use. Cortisone-type drugs are now reserved for patients who have failed to respond to less potent medicines such as those already mentioned. When used, cortisone-type drugs are often combined with other medicines so as to allow the patient to have smaller doses of the cortisone drug. This, in turn, decreases the likelihood of the patient developing any of the multitude of side effects including thinning of the skin, skin hemorrhages, cataracts, stomach ulcers, bone softening, weight gain, and increased susceptibility to infection.

The major complications attributed to cortisone drugs occur in patients who take this medication for periods of months to years. Short courses of treatment are less dangerous, as are shots of cortisone spaced at long intervals. In contrast to the pill or shot given into the system, cortisone injection into joints does not have the risks mentioned above. Instead, the good and bad effects are limited to the injected joint. The good effect is immediate relief of inflammation in many patients. The only immediately serious side effect is accidental infection of a joint during introduction of the needle. Repeated injection of the same joint may, however, lead to cartilage destruction.

Even though serious side effects are well recognized in cortisone-treated patients, its use has allowed many otherwise disabled people to be more mobile, and, therefore, more productive members of society. The drug is most effective in rheumatoid arthritis and its sister diseases such as lupus erythematosus, and in any form of arthritis except infectious arthritis, if injected directly into the joint. Cortisone is not useful in osteoarthritis and gout if given in the pill form.

The various preparations of cortisone and its synthetic derivatives are too numerous to mention. The most common ones include Prednisone, which is marketed under many brand names: Medrol (Prednisolone), Decadron (Dexamethasone), and Kenalog and Aristocort (Triamcinolone).

Medications in Arthritis

ANTI-CANCER DRUGS.

Drugs originally developed for use in leukemia and other forms of cancer have been found to be of use in rheumatoid arthritis and some of its sister diseases, notably lupus erythematosus and polyarteritis. These compounds are very powerful, with potentially fatal side effects. They must, therefore, be reserved for only the most severely affected patients. Even in these patients, all the other available forms of therapy should be tried before anti-cancer drugs are considered. Patients taking these drugs must be carefully watched by their doctors so that serious side effects can be quickly identified and treated.

This group of drugs includes Cytoxan (Cyclophosphamide), Imuran (Azathioprine), Purinethol (6-Mercaptopurine), Leukeran (Chlorambucil), and Methotrexate.

ANTI-GOUT DRUGS

The drugs used in the treatment of gout may be divided into two general types. There are those drugs aimed at the treatment of the acute attack with its attendant pain, and those drugs whose job it is to lower the uric acid in the body. These latter drugs are of value in preventing future attacks, but are not meant to be helpful for the pain of any single attack.

The drugs used in the acute attack include Indocin and Butazolidin, which have already been mentioned, and Colchicine. Colchicine, a plant derivative, was found to

87

be effective in treating acute gout attacks many centuries ago. It is still used in gout, but is somewhat inconvenient to use and often causes mild bothersome side effects. Colchicine is not of value in any of the other common types of arthritis. In the typical gout patient, these drugs are needed only during acute attacks. The drugs used to lower uric acid in the body are also unique to gout, since lowering of the uric acid (as measured in the blood) is not beneficial to other forms of arthritis. These uric-acid-lowering drugs may also be divided into two types. Benemid (Probenecid) and Anturane (Sulfinpyrazone) work by causing the excess uric acid to be excreted by the kidneys. Zyloprim (Allopurinol), the other type, stops the body from making excessive amounts of uric acid. Benemid, Anturane, and Zyloprim have relatively few side effects. They may occasionally cause nausea or rash. One common side effect is the development of an acute gout attack during the first few weeks of treatment with these drugs. This is probably due to shifting of uric acid in gouty joints as the uric acid level drops. Once started, the uric-acid-lowering agents should be continued indefinitely because the possibility of repeated gout attacks exists for the lifetime of the patient.

ANALGESICS

Analgesics (painkillers) are not specific treatment for arthritis, but they are frequently used to help relieve pain in arthritis. Propoxyphene (Darvon and SK-65), Talwin, and codeine-containing medications may be safely used in association with other arthritis medicine. Analgesics alone should probably not be used in arthritis except in very unusual circumstances. Habit-forming painkillers should be avoided since arthritis is often chronic in nature and the use of such medications could lead to addiction.

MUSCLE RELAXANTS

Since muscular pain may be a prominent feature of arthritic conditions, muscle-relaxing medications may be of value. In particular, tendonitis is basically a muscular problem and may respond well to these drugs. Muscle relaxants include Equagesic, Parafon, Robaxin, Norflex, and Soma. Tranquilizers such as Valium and Librium are also effective muscle relaxants.

EXPERIMENTAL DRUGS

There are literally dozens of experimental drugs being researched in arthritis. Many of these drugs are similar to the ones recently approved for use in this country. Others are more potent compounds.

Of the more potent drugs, Penicillamine has been used extensively in Great Britain with promising results. Penicillamine is well known in the United States for its use in Wilson's disease, which is an inherited condition involving abnormal copper metabolism. In rheumatoid arthritis (where no copper metabolism problems are known) this drug has been found effective in many patients who have failed to respond to standard forms of treatment. Many arthritis specialists in the United States have been experimenting with Penicillamine.

Medications in Arthritis

In conclusion, the selection of any medication for arthritis treatment is the responsibility of your physician. In determining the most effective drug for your particular condition, he will need your cooperation in following his orders and in giving him an honest account of your reactions, whether good or bad. He needs this information to know what is best for you. Do not experiment on your own or with drugs which promise dramatic results or cures.

CHAPTER SEVEN

Alternatives in Pain Control and Relaxation

The importance of pain control in the management of arthritis should not be underestimated. The presence of pain greatly contributes to joint immobility and contracture, muscle spasm, and atrophy. If pain is insufficiently controlled, the person with arthritis is likely to become increasingly immobile because it hurts so much to move about. Avoidance of social activities and even failure to perform personal care such as hair brushing, shaving, and bathing may become an acceptable way of life for the arthritic who must deal with constant pain.

A few patients develop a "chronic pain personality," which is generally characterized by some degree of drug dependency, use of pain to manipulate family and friends, and loss of true motivation toward a treatment program. Physicians and other health care workers are faced with an almost impossible task when they attempt to treat such a patient with traditional methods of pain relief. Frustration and misunderstanding may develop, with deterioration of the professional-patient relationship. The anguished patient may then begin roaming from one doctor to another, from one clinic to another—a journey that is always expensive and generally unrewarding. This patient becomes a prime target for quacks who prey on persons who are desperately searching for relief from the chronic pain they often live with each day.

What is pain? Most certainly, it is a sensation with a degree of intensity known only to the individual patient. It has been shown to be affected by environmental and psychological factors. Although pain is almost always physical at the onset, emotions can quickly become involved. Some health care workers feel that if pain can be well controlled when it first occurs, many of the psychological problems associated with pain which greatly complicate treatment can be avoided.

Pain is an accurate warning mechanism which signals that the body has experienced trauma or malfunction. It is, therefore, a valuable diagnostic tool in determining the nature and severity of injury or illness.

We feel pain only after the pain message has traveled from the site of irritation to the brain. The pain message travels along a network of nerves to the spinal cord and finally up to the brain. Then, when the pain message is interpretted by the brain, pain is actually felt as a body sensation. Traditional therapies for pain control—chemical, physical, surgical, and psychiatric—are all methods of interrupting the pain message before it is recognized by the brain. In addition to these traditional therapies, several promising new methods of controlling chronic pain have recently been investigated. Two of these, transcutaneous nerve stimulation and biofeedback, warrant discussion here because of their potentially significant value in treating pain which accompanies arthritis and in helping the patient to learn to monitor and control his muscle activity.

Within the past few years, the fields of electronics and bioengineering have given the medical profession an innovative approach to pain control, which is called TNS, or transcutaneous nerve stimulation. Although the use of electrical current passed into the body to relieve pain is as old as Hippocrates, it was not until quite recently that the

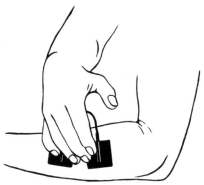

Figure 25. TNS nerve stimulator.

medical community once again became interested in the use of electrical stimulation as a method of altering transmission of impulses through the nerve pathways.

The transcutaneous nerve stimulator is a small battery-operated generator with two or four electrodes. The electrodes are taped to the skin over the painful area or at selected sites close to the spinal column. When the unit is turned on, an electrical current passes between the electrodes, and if successful, masks or covers up the sensation of pain. By stimulating the nerve fibers, the electrical current blocks the transmission of pain messages before they reach the brain. The exact mechanism of this interruption is not yet known, but is under investigation.

The duration and intensity of the electrical stimulation is controlled by the patient by means of a small, box-like unit worn on a belt around his waist. The pain is relieved by low-level intensities of electrical stimulation which the patient generally finds comfortable or does not feel at all. The electrodes must be cleaned frequently and reapplied to the appropriate area by the patient or family member in order to insure proper transmission of the electrical current to the skin and to prevent irritation of the skin under the electrodes.

A physician's prescription is necessary to purchase the electrical stimulator. The patient is taught by a physical therapist or nurse how to place the electrodes properly and operate the unit. The patient does not have to be hospitalized in order to receive instruction for using his unit; however, many physicians and technicians feel that the patient may benefit from a brief hospital stay, during which he can receive thorough instructions without distraction.

Successful pain control with the stimulator depends to a great extent on the patient's attitude and the skill and diligence of the instructor in placing the electrodes and teaching the patient how to use the unit. Initially, the patient uses the electrical stimulator twenty-four hours a day. Some patients obtain significant pain relief immediately, while others may need several days. After one or two months, the patient may find that he obtains adequate pain relief with eight hours or less of stimulation. Some patients find that five to ten minutes of stimulation in the morning permits satisfactory relief from pain for the rest of the day. Or electrical stimulation may be used only at night to obtain a restful sleep, free from the dull, nagging aches in hip or knee joints which can be particularly bothersome at night.

At this time, no significant side effects have been encountered in patients using the transcutaneous nerve stimulator. Some have used it for several years and continue to experience no problems.

The transcutaneous nerve stimulator has been effective in the management of back and neck pain associated with joints of the arm and leg. One electrode placed on each side of an affected joint may lessen the arthritic pain. Electrodes which have been strategically placed on the shoulder and/or arm may relieve pain in the arm, hand, and fingers. Migraine and tension headaches, which often accompany chronic ailments and prevent relaxation, may be helped by placing the electrodes high on the back of the neck. By experimenting with various placements, the instructor can pinpoint the placements which help the particular patient most.

The arthritic patient must be especially carefully instructed when given the transcutaneous nerve stimulator. He must monitor the ongoing process of his disease by being constantly aware of increased swelling, redness, temperature, and pain. These are indications that an acute inflammatory battle is raging in the joint, and such a joint must be carefully protected and sometimes even immobilized until the acute reaction has subsided. Failure to do so may result in further destruction and deformity of the joint. If the transcutaneous nerve stimulator is being used for pain control at such an acutely inflamed joint, the patient must be careful to curtail activity and weight-bearing of the joint even though he may feel little or no pain.

Proper joint protection principles must still be heeded. For example, if electrical stimulation is being used to relieve low back pain, the patient must still continue to maintain good posture and must observe caution when lifting and carrying objects. If the stimulator is used to relieve hip joint pain, it may still be necessary for the patient to use crutches in order to prevent further deformity and degeneration of the hip joint. This is particularly true if he is overweight.

Some patients experience complete pain relief while others gain only partial relief. One researcher estimates that approximately 55-60 percent of all patients using the unit gain enough relief to allow a cutback in their daily pain medication. However, the patient should never stop using any anti-inflammatory agents prescribed by his physician, unless his physician advises him to do so. If the arthritis patient is not able to learn that he still must restrict activity when necessary, observe joint protection principles, and continue taking necessary medications, then he probably is not a good candidate for a transcutaneous nerve stimulator. Such a person may need to experience pain as a signal to prompt him to deal properly with his disease.

In this discussion of the potential value of transcutaneous nerve stimulation in arthritis, we do not want to imply that it is a miraculous new agent which can cure arthritis. As we have said many times, there is no cure for arthritis. However, some of the techniques being developed to treat chronic pain do have merit, and although some patients are not helped by transcutaneous nerve stimulation, it is another tool which the physician may recommend for the patient who has not been sufficiently helped by the traditional therapies.

The other new technique which may be helpful to arthritics, although in ways different from the pain control possible with transcutaneous nerve stimulation, is the use of biofeedback. Biofeedback is a process for learning voluntary control over internal body functions which were previously thought to be involuntary or uncontrollable. Biofeedback provides the patient with signals which he can hear or see. His internal responses are picked up by electrodes taped to his skin, transmitted to the biofeedback unit as electrical impulses, and then translated into a sound or light he can observe. This process gives him continuous information about his body functions such as heart rate, blood pressure, muscle tension, and skin temperature. This information is then used by the patient to learn to control at will his internal responses. Although little biofeedback research has been done to date specifically with arthritics, much has been done in areas such as relaxation training, pain control, hand-warming, and muscle re-education. Since these areas are of concern to many arthritics, biofeedback may offer some arthritics help in re-educating the body to respond differently.

Biofeedback training is becoming increasingly useful in teaching relaxation. Most chronic diseases including arthritis are almost always accompanied by nervousness and tension. Insomnia, severe headache, reduced ability to concentrate, facial grimaces, abnormal excitability of the heart and lungs, muscle tremor, excessive and loud talking, fidgeting, and increased reaction to sudden or loud noise or other stimuli are often manifestations of high levels of anxiety. Some medical professionals who work with chronically ill patients have recognized the importance of treating these anxiety symptoms in an effort to more effectively manage the initial disease process.

For relaxation training, the patient is placed in a semi-dark room in a comfortable chair or recliner. The electrodes of the biofeedback instrument are placed on his forehead over the muscles which "knit" the brow. The tension or activity of these muscles has been shown to be a good indication of the tension levels of the entire body. Forearm and back neck muscles may also be used to monitor tension levels in this way.

After the electrodes are in place on the skin directly over the muscle, the patient is instructed by the technician to contract these muscles, then relax. With contraction of the muscles, the patient may hear a loud or rapidly repeating tone. When the muscles relax, the volume or rate of the tone diminishes. The biofeedback instrument acts much like a stethoscope which allows the doctor to hear heart sounds. Biofeedback allows the patient to "hear" his own muscle activity.

The immediate goal of relaxation training is to utilize the biofeedback instrument to obtain the lowest tone volume or rate possible, which indicates a low level of muscle contraction. After the initial instruction by the technician, it becomes the patient's responsibility to learn to control the biofeedback signal and thus his own muscle tension. He must practice the relaxation techniques at home and gradually wean himself from the instrument. The ultimate goal of biofeedback training has been reached when the patient is capable of identifying the onset of increasing stress, pain, and anxiety symptoms and successfully interrupts or subdues these symptoms by utilizing the relaxation training without the aid of the biofeedback signals. When this happens, it indicates that the patient has learned to successfully control his anxiety in the environment within which it is originating, which is usually the job or home.

Biofeedback training for relaxation may be facilitated by teaching the patient to use Jacobson's Progressive Relaxation Exercises (see Glossary), which allow him to compare or become aware of the difference in feeling between a fully tensed and a fully relaxed muscle. One of the reasons some patients are unable to relax even though they are trying very hard to do so is that they are unable to make this distinction. Thus, they think that a muscle is relaxed when it is not. Another method of helping patients to relax is to play a pre-recorded tape which provides autosuggestions and other verbal stimuli to help the patient find the kind of thoughts and mental pictures which help him relax. Abdominal breathing exercises also promote relaxation and are easily learned.

It can be seen that biofeedback provides a means of helping persons to change or control the way they typically respond to various stimuli by increased muscle tension. While biofeedback does not alter or treat the underlying causes of such stress and tension, the patient can benefit by knowing that he can control his body responses, and can learn more appropriate ways of dealing with tension.

Like transcutaneous nerve stimulation, biofeedback training should be only a part of a total treatment program. Relaxation training has been used in conjunction with psychiatric counseling, marital and vocational counseling, and physical therapy and other measures which are aimed at identifying and resolving the source of the anxiety or pain problem.

Relaxation training has been used successfully in the treatment of anxiety reactions, insomnia, migraine-tension headaches, pain control, and stress reduction, any or all of which may accompany chronic illness. The arthritic can benefit from relaxation training by learning cues which indicate tension build-up in his muscles, which in turn can be exaggerated by tension, fear, and anxiety. The end result of this tension process is joint pain and stiffness, which lead to more pain. Interrupting this cycle before it becomes well established is the major contribution of relaxation training to arthritis management.

For the arthritic, biofeedback training may also be helpful in increasing skin temperature of the hands and feet. By utilizing autosuggestion with biofeedback, some individuals have learned to raise the skin temperature of their fingers and hands by as much as three to ten degrees, and consequently relieve pain, numbness, and tingling in their fingers. Most persons who have successfully accomplished this report increased flexibility and ability to perform hand activities more easily.

Heat-sensitive electrodes are placed on the skin of the hands or fingers and the patient is asked to repeat phrases such as, "my hands and arms are heavy and warm" and "warmth is flowing into my hands, they are warm, warm, warm...." As the electrodes pick up changes in skin temperature, this information is fed back to the patient by signals from the biofeedback unit to assist him in learning to alter skin temperature consistently. This type of training has been used predominately in the treatment of Raynaud's Disease, which is a disorder of the blood vessels characterized by acute attacks during which the hands become very painful, cold, and bluish in color. Success in increasing hand function and decreasing pain has been reported by many researchers. Some reports indicate that this kind of temperature training is also beneficial for arthritics with hand involvement which limits flexibility and function.

Biofeedback has been extremely promising in the area of muscle re-education. For those patients who have lost the use of muscles due to paralysis or lack of use, biofeedback offers a workable, precise method of learning how to restore voluntary muscle function and regain purposeful movement.

The biofeedback instrument gives the patient information about how much work a particular muscle is actually doing, or if in fact the muscle is working at all during an exercise session. Biofeedback does not in itself strengthen the muscle; it can only provide clues to the patient about the amount of activity of a muscle and the type of effort and exercises which produce more activity in that muscle.

Biofeedback training for muscle re-education is usually undertaken in a physical therapy clinic and supervised by a physician or physical therapist. The patient is placed in a relaxed position in a quiet, isolated room. The electrodes may first be placed on a "good" muscle to teach the patient how to use the biofeedback signals. Then the electrodes are placed on the skin over the malfunctioning muscle. The therapist may then demonstrate the movement which will elicit the desired muscle response, and the patient is asked to attempt to repeat this motion. By means of the biofeedback signals, the patient is able to see or hear the amount of activity his effort produced. The electrodes are left in place during the exercise session so that the patient is constantly informed about the results of his efforts including the type, amount, and duration of effort needed to strengthen the muscle and restore voluntary control over it. This process may be indicated for the arthritic who has markedly weak muscles and has essentially forgotten how to make them respond at will.

The concept of biofeedback destroys the idea that healing the body and restoring function and health is the sole responsibility of the health professionals. For the first time, the patient is given the opportunity to assume the greatest amount of responsibility and direction for his own treatment and restoration to health. The result is seen not only in his obtaining relief from his physical problems, but also in improvement in his attitude toward treatment. When the chronically ill person learns that he really can control what is happening within his body, he gains confidence in his ability to be an active, equal partner with professionals who are treating him. A dramatic improvement is often noticed and recovery is speeded. Rather than give the patient a lecture about how his mental attitude and strong will can influence the course of his illness, biofeedback provides recognizable evidence that he is in control of his body and emotions, enabling him to see the interdependency of body and mind that cannot be ignored if a treatment program is to be effective.

CHAPTER EIGHT

Surgical Repair in Arthritis

Great advances have been made recently in surgical procedures used for rheumatic diseases. One of the most promising types of surgery for the more severely involved patient is the total joint replacement; however, constant improvements in other types of procedures have rendered them more effective also, so that the orthopedic surgeon now has quite a wide range of choices when surgery is indicated.

The primary aims of surgery in arthritis are: 1) to relieve pain, 2) to increase or restore function, and 3) to prevent destruction of other joints. In selecting a particular procedure, the surgeon must consider factors such as the patient's age, his life style, the type of arthritis, and the extent and type of joint damage. While surgery is not limited to patients with osteoarthritis and rheumatoid arthritis, these two conditions comprise the majority of rheumatic conditions in which surgery is utilized.

Surgery can be used selectively both in problems originating in the synovium, as in persons with rheumatoid arthritis, and in mechanical problems such as those encountered in persons with degenerative joint disease.

Basically, surgery becomes necessary in some case of osteoarthritis because the articular cartilage has been severely damaged. Cartilage degeneration is thought to be caused by the interaction of nutritive, mechanical, and chemical mechanisms. Abnormal stress may rupture the joint membranes and degeneration of the joint surfaces follows. Enzymes which are released as a result of this degeneration further deteriorate the joint tissues and the joint becomes more susceptible to further mechanical damage. A vicious cycle which leads to progressive damage is thus indicated.

As has been stated previously, the cause of rheumatoid arthritis is unknown, although several theories have been advanced. Whatever the cause, surgery may be indicated in cases where joint destruction has led to pain and deformity which interfere significantly with the patient's ability to function.

Except in cases where surgery is used to correct malalignment or prevent destruction of other joints, it is used only after conservative measures such as medication and physical therapy have failed.

The types of surgery performed in arthritis can be classified according to purpose as either therapeutic or salvage. Therapeutic procedures may be used in patients where degenerative disease is present but some cartilage remains in part or all of the joint. The object of therapeutic procedures is to relieve the abnormal force concentrations that have caused the damage to occur and to give the cartilage a chance to repair itself. This can be accomplished in some instances by transferring the load of weight-bearing from one part of the involved joint to another. Salvage surgery is the name given to procedures used when all or nearly all of the joint cartilage has been lost. Fusions and total joint replacements often fall into this category.

The surgical procedures most commonly performed are described below:

1. *Synovectomy.* In this procedure, the synovium is removed. The surgery is often used to relieve pain in rheumatoid arthritis. Best results are obtained if done early in the course of the disease, after medical therapy has failed but before much cartilage destruction has occurred. Age is rarely a contraindication, nor is the general activity of the rheumatoid arthritis, so long as the patient is well enough to undergo surgery.

2. *Osteotomy.* Any surgical cutting of bone can be termed an osteotomy. The main role of osteotomy in arthritis is to correct malalignment, which involves shifting the weight-bearing to a new part of the joint. The procedure often is performed to correct deformities which may be due to flexion contracture, which is inability to straighten the joint. It is most effective if the flexion contracture does not exceed 30°. Figure 26 shows a knee joint realigned by removal of a wedge of bone.

Osteotomy is not recommended for cases where only a small amount of joint cartilage remains or where advanced disease or severe joint destruction is evident. It is used in both osteoarthritis and rheumatoid arthritis, but more commonly in osteoarthritis. Osteotomy does not

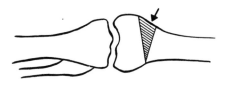

Figure 26. Removal of the wedge will allow the bone to be realigned and redistributed more evenly.

alter the activity of the disease in rheumatoid arthritis. Age is no contraindication to osteotomy; however, hip osteotomy is seldom performed on patients over sixty with degenerative joint disease because a total hip replacement is usually preferable.

3. *Capsulectomy and tenotomy.* This operation is used in cases where flexion contracture exceeds 30°, but may also be used to correct such contractures of less than 30° where osteotomy would not be suitable. A capsulectomy should not be carried out in cases of severe joint destruc-

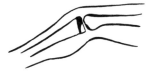

Figure 27 a. The wedge of bone (dark area) to be removed.

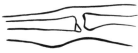

Figure 27 b. The realigned joint. In order to perform the osteotomy, the joint capsule must first be removed and the tendon cut.

tion. The capsulectomy consists of removing the joint capsule; the tenotomy is the cutting of the tendon. Figures 27a and 27b show the results of an osteotomy which included a capsulectomy and tenotomy.

4. *Arthroplasty.* An arthroplasty consists of placing a metallic or plastic surface between the existing joint surfaces. It is effective in more severe cases of both osteoarthritis and rheumatoid arthritis. The three most commonly used devices are the mold, cup, and total replacement. The term "mold" describes a prothesis designed to oppose a new joint surface rather than to replace the joint. The mold is made of vitallium or other metallic compound. Permanent results have not been particularly good, and the procedure is rarely used today. The "cup" is just that—a cup-shaped device which fits over the head of the femur and meets the acetabulum. The cup arthroplasty is used primarily today in young persons or when current or potential infection indicates that a total replacement would give less than optimal results. The differences among the three types of prostheses can be seen in Figures 28a, b, and c.

The total hip replacement has offered one of the most dramatic procedures ever to be performed in terms of ability of the patient to move about and regain function that was lost. The total hip replacement has come to be preferred to the cup arthroplasty for a variety of reasons including: 1) superior pain relief, 2) increased functional capacity, 3) greater reliability, 4) shorter recovery period, and 5) ability to correct discrepancies in leg length.

The total joint replacement has been used now for about a decade. The most common sites for such surgery

Figure 28a. Mold for knee.

Figure 28b. Acetabular cup for hip joint.

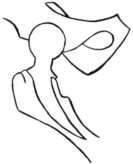

Figure 28c. Total replacement prosthesis shown in place in hip joint.

in order of importance and frequency are: hip, knee, ankle, fingers and carpal bones, and wrist.

The prostheses are made of metallic compounds of cobalt, chromium, and molybdenum, or of polyethylene. Dr. John Charnley developed a widely-used procedure using a polyethylene prosthesis and an acrylic cement called methyl methacrylate. This cement provides a precise fit, which distributes the load more evenly. There is an overall infection rate of less than 1 percent from all causes in joint replacement procedures. One of the major drawbacks in using total joint replacements is that they are so new that it is not yet known for certain just how long they will last. For this reason, some physicians feel that the procedure should not be used on young persons.

Silastic prostheses are flexible but cannot withstand as much stress as the metallic type. They are used primarily for persons with rheumatoid arthritis of the fingers and wrists. While a full 90° range of motion is not generally possible, considerable function can be restored.

5. *Arthrodesis.* An arthrodesis is a fusion; the joint is permanently immoilized by insertion of a metallic nail or piece of bone taken from elsewhere in the body. In rheumatoid arthritis, it may be used if a total joint arthroplasty has failed. There can be major surgical complications including increased danger of infection.

The surgeon must carefully weigh the potential harmful effects of an arthrodesis against the benefits and make a choice based on the factors previously mentioned. For example, if an arthrodesis is performed, the patient's employment opportunities can be limited, especially if the job entails driving, bending, and other activities where flexibility is required. Social activities such as dancing and attending movies also may be curtailed. Needless to say, dressing can also be extremely difficult. As you can see, not only health needs, but social and economic considerations will also affect the surgeon's selection of procedure.

Special problems are posed by the patient with lack of motivation to undergo surgery even though he really needs it, and by the patient who has many joints involved with rheumatoid arthritis. The patient who lacks motivation for surgery may prefer to remain handicapped for a variety of reasons, such as being very fearful of any type of surgery, using his disability to control or manipulate others, or simply feeling so depressed and defeated that he doesn't want to exert any effort to improve his condition. Psychological counseling may be indicated for such a patient. For that matter, counseling may be beneficial to anyone contemplating major surgery. It can help lay fears to rest, prevent unrealistic expectations of results of the procedure, and can also help the patient make a satisfactory adjustment after the surgery. Some of the problems faced in working with the patient with multiple joint involvement have been touched on previously. Such a patient may be very apprehensive and the surgeon may be hard-pressed literally to know where to begin with someone who could be helped by several different operations. However, if the patient is in fairly good general health and has a positive outlook, chances for satisfactory results from surgery are enhanced considerably.

Insofar as results of surgery in arthritis are concerned, several studies give insight into long-term results with significant numbers of patients. A United States study of over 6,500 surgical cases involving a variety of procedures used on rheumatoid arthritis patients showed that less that 2.5 percent developed complications of any kind. A long-term study in Switzerland of 2,200 patients who had undergone hip osteotomies for degenerative joint disease revealed that after periods ranging from five to twelve years, 30 percent were painfree and 53 percent had reduced pain; 60 percent had increased ability to walk.

Evaluations in this study were subjective, based on the patient's reports, but indicate a high level of satisfaction with the procedures after several years. This small sampling of the many studies done on arthritis surgery shows that it is relatively safe and yields good results.

As with any treatment for arthritis, the physician's advice should be heeded. If you feel that surgery may help your arthritic condition, you should discuss it with your physician, who can explain his reasons for recommending it or advising you against it. Remember that your arthritis is not exactly like anyone else's and so the treatment your physician recommends most likely will not be like your neighbor's or friend's or relative's. However, if he does recommend surgery, there is no reason not to feel confident that your recovery will be prompt and the results good.

CHAPTER NINE

The Importance of Nutrition in Arthritis

Many diets have been promoted as preventive or curative for arthritis. However, at this time there is no scientific evidence that any particular diet can do either. Until proof that there is a direct link between nutrition and arthritis has been established, the arthritis patient would be wise to disregard such claims.

The fact that in arthritis there may be alternating periods of remission, or disappearance of symptoms, and flare-ups can deceive us into believing that whatever diet we happened to be following at that particular time was responsible for the remission. If an arthritis patient who is following a treatment program which combines medication, exercise, and perhaps some other modalities known to be helpful in treating arthritis then also tries a new diet, it is difficult to know which of the treatments is helping or not. That is not to say that good nutrition has nothing to offer the arthritis patient, however. Good nutrition plays a significant part in general good health and well-being by enabling the body to fight off infections, supplying adequate energy for the tasks we want to perform, repairing damage, and accomplishing many other vital tasks in the various body systems.

What is good nutrition? There is no one authoritative guide to good nutrition which everyone should automatically follow. Nevertheless, although each person's body is different and utilizes food in a slightly different manner than another's, it is safe to generalize within certain limits. A person who has not had extensive gastric surgery or metabolic disease and is not in the immediate post-operative stage can probably be considered average and follow the guidelines which have been set up for normal nutritional requirements. In developing a sound individual nutrition program, each person also must take into account his customary activity level; a person who participates actively in sports or performs heavy physical labor will usually need more calories and nutrients than a person who is relatively inactive.

First of all, let's examine what the average person needs for good nutrition. Many scientific studies have been conducted over the years on the need for protein, vitamins, minerals, and other elements in the diet. As research and measurement techniques become more sophisticated and accurate and our knowledge of the human body increases, we find that adjustments have been made in the amounts of nutrients recommended by experts in order to maintain good health. As a result, we now see the MDR, or minimum daily requirement, listed on an increasing number of the foods we purchase. The

The Importance of Nutrition in Arthritis

MDR was established after much research as the lowest amount of each particular nutritional substance required by the average person to maintain body functions without symptoms of nutritional deficiency. If we are consuming a balanced diet and no deficiencies are apparent, we can assume that we are receiving an adequate amount of the required nutrients. However, some of us may require supplemental amounts of certain nutrients because of acute or chronic illness or inability of the body to utilize a particular substance. While symptoms of the more common deficiencies are known to most of us, we need professional advice to diagnose exactly which substances in what amounts are lacking. The physician may be able to diagnose certain conditions on the basis of a patient history and/or observation, or he may order laboratory tests which can help him to accurately diagnose such disorders. Self-diagnosis and treatment is extremely risky because many disorders unrelated to nutrition have symptoms similar to those caused by certain nutritional deficiencies. Only qualified professionals should prescribe large doses of supplements, because some substances can be toxic if taken in large amounts. In addition to being toxic, over-utilization of supplemental vitamins, called hypervitaminosis, can actually lower resistance to infection and cause damage to susceptible parts of the body such as the liver and kidneys.

Many diet plans which have been published in books and magazines claim that certain foods or supplements will help relieve or cure specific diseases or build up a specific part of the body. These diets are not to be recommended.

The Importance of Nutrition in Arthritis

The following table shows amounts of various foods needed daily for good nutrition for the average adult. Protein, mineral, and vitamin needs of the average person will be met by this plan.

DAILY FOOD GUIDE

Milk group	*2 cups or more*
Meat group	*2 or more servings* Count as one serving: 3 oz. lean cooked meat, poultry, or fish without bone—or 2 eggs—or 1 cup cooked dry beans, peas, lentils.
Vegetable-fruit group	*4 or more servings* Include daily: 1 serving of citrus fruit & 1 serving dark-green or deep-yellow vegetable and 2 or more servings other vegetables and fruits.
Bread-cereal group	*4 or more servings* Count as one serving: 1 slice bread, 1 oz. ready-to-eat cereal, ½ cup cooked cereal, macaroni, or rice.

116

The Importance of Nutrition in Arthritis

In addition to simply needing certain nutrients, our bodies must have some in specific combinations in order to manufacture other essential nutrients within the body. That is to say, one substance can act as a catalyst or starter, enabling our bodies to make needed nutrients from the various raw materials we eat. For example, vitamin C helps the body to utilize the B vitamins, and vitamin D is important in calcium absorption.

It seems a paradox that a person can be suffering from under-nutrition, yet be over-eating. But a person can be consuming too many "empty" calories from foods which contain low amounts of nutrients and high amounts of calories. A certain portion of the calories we consume is used in maintaining basic body functions such as breathing and digestion. To this must be added enough calories to sustain our usual level of activity. Any excess over this amount is converted to fat and stored in the body tissues. We see 900 calorie per day diets, 1500 calorie per day diets, and all sorts of charts on how to calculate the number of calories in foods. While we can use average height and weight tables to estimate the number of calories we need, experience may be the most important factor in determining our calorie requirements. If we are within 10 percent of our desirable weight and our weight is relatively stable over time, we probably are taking in an adequate number of calories. If we are overweight or underweight, the only effective long-term treatment is re-education in eating habits. It is important that a physician be consulted before attempting to either gain or lose a significant amount. Persons with any acute or chronic condition such as arthritis should be especially careful to avoid fad diets or crash weight loss techniques such as fasting. Fasting should be undertaken only under a physician's supervision, and diuretics and other weight loss aids should be taken only if prescribed by a physician.

Many persons are surprised when they begin to gain weight after about age 35 or 40. While the effects of aging are highly individual, studies have shown that the average person needs about 25 percent fewer calories from middle age on than when in his twenties. Much of this reduction is due to actual loss of body cells after growth ceases, which is usually at about age 20. The lean body mass decreases and the amount of body fat increases from age 25 on. A good and easy way to learn exactly what your eating habits are is to write down everything you eat or drink for several days immediately after eating it, including between-meal snacks and drinks. Then, with the help of a guide which shows the number of calories in various foods and the Daily Food Guide above, you can make a fairly accurate estimate of whether you are getting the various nutrients you need and maintaining an appropriate calorie intake. If excessive calorie intake is a problem, modifications can be made which will reduce calories while still ensuring that enough nutrients are eaten. For example, skim milk can be substituted for whole milk; poultry or fish can be eaten more often than the fattier red meats; rich sauces can be eliminated. Excellent cookbooks are available which can guide you in planning and preparing nutritious meals within your daily calorie requirement.

For persons who have difficulty preparing meals for themselves, programs such as Meals on Wheels can be very helpful. For a moderate fee per meal, a well-prepared, nutritionally sound hot meal is delivered to your home. Special diets are usually available, also.

For the person who can get out and about and enjoys companionship at lunch-time on occasion, many church and civic groups serve low-cost, nutritious meals at various locations in many cities nationwide. For the temporarily homebound arthritic, services including meal preparation are often available through local homemaker or home health services agencies. A sliding fee is usually available for those on limited incomes.

Besides requiring fewer calories as we grow older, we find that digestive functioning decreases. There is a reduction in muscle tone of the stomach, intestines, and colon. There also is a reduction of volume, acidity, and pepsin content of the gastric juices. This reduced acidity may lead to poor calcium and iron absorption, and the decreased muscle activity may lead to constipation, especially if insufficient fluids and fiber are consumed. Because the digestive process is not so efficient, many older persons may tend to over-use anti-acids, which can lead to chemical imbalance and further aggravate symptoms of indigestion.

The person with rheumatoid arthritis may find that he has special nutritional needs. The anemia which often accompanies RA is not necessarily due to a lack of iron in the blood. It may result, instead, from interference with the body's utilization of its iron stores, blocking production of hemoglobin and other blood substances. This can occur in the active phase of RA when inflammation and other symptoms are present. The physician must pre-

119

scribe the type and amount of iron needed on an individual basis.

Some researchers have found that increased nutritional needs occur in rheumatic arthritis patients. Since nutritional needs vary widely on an individual basis when dealing with any kind of disease, often only a physician with training and experience in treating that specific family of disorders can prescribe the proper dietary management program which will bring about the desired results. A competent and conscientious physician will not hesitate to request a consultation with others, such as dietitians, who may be more knowledgeable than he when problems he cannot adequately manage arise.

Another problem, which some persons mistakenly believe is a type of arthritis, is osteoporosis. Researchers have found that calcium deficiency in older women can lead to osteoporosis, which in turn is aggravated by hormone insufficiency. In osteoporosis, adequate amounts of vitamin D must also be taken, because of its importance in calcium absorption. Dietary studies have shown that adequate amounts of calcium are often not consumed by older persons, so it is not surprising that many older women show symptoms of osteoporosis. A physician can advise the osteoporosis patient as to precautions to be taken and special nutritional needs she may have.

In summation, we want to stress that basic good nutrition is very important to everyone, whether he has arthritis or not. Any nutritional problems should be referred to a physician, who can diagnose the cause of your particular symptoms and recommend treatment.

The Importance of Nutrition in Arthritis

Fad diets and claims that certain diets or foods can cure or prevent rheumatic conditions, including arthritis, should be disregarded.

CHAPTER TEN

Communicating with Your Professional Health Worker

In preparing this series of instructions, we have considered topics which would be informative, interesting, and practical for the person afflicted with arthritis who is sincerely concerned with following a comprehensive treatment program. The assessment of a patient's adjustment to a chronic illness is not complete with merely a medical evaluation. Joint symptoms may have decreased and the patient may be physically improved, yet his anxiety, hostility, and inability to accept the disease may constitute a continuing problem for the patient and for those with whom he is associated. Now we would like to explore the area of communication, limiting our discussion to the interrelationships a patient has with his professional worker: physician, physical therapist, nurse, and other trained technicians.

First of all, let's examine what communication is. The best definition we've come across is, "Communication is the relationship which is set up by transmitting and receiving a message." We must realize that both the sender and the receiver bring to the relationship several factors that influence the relationship: his communication skills, his attitudes, his knowledge, and his experiences as a member of a social system and a particular culture. When we look at this list of potential barriers to effective communication, it's a wonder that anything good happens when we attempt to communicate!

As we all know, "body-language" or non-verbal messages add another complication to our attempts to communicate effectively. We've all had a confusing experience where someone's expression or actions contradicted his words, and we consequently received a garbled message. Unfortunately, some of us are unaware of sending double messages, and as a result, we constantly have problems in communicating. Keep in mind that both spoken and body language affect each situation where we are trying to communicate.

Let's now look at the relationships we have with physicians and other health care personnel and try to identify ways we can improve communication.

When illness strikes, the logical beginning is a visit to the doctor. Now let's set up an ideal doctor-patient relationship: We will assume that your symptoms cause you to suspect arthritis, and that you have selected a reputable doctor whose education and experience make him well qualified in this field. We will further assume that he will order a complete and thorough physical examination and any laboratory tests, X-rays, or other measures which can help him to make an accurate diagnosis. Having diagnosed arthritis and having determined the form, i.e., osteoarthritis, rheumatoid, gout, or other, he must then communicate his findings to you, the patient.

Informing a patient that he has a disease for which there is no cure requires great sensitivity and skill. The patient's knowledge may be scanty or erroneous. What little he does know probably reinforces rather than dispels his fear and anxiety. Misinformation from friends and fear-provoking articles convince the arthritis patient that he can do little to prevent pain and deformity and that he will eventually become a total invalid. These fears are often due to ignorance of the natural course of chronic arthritis. If a patient doesn't understand the nature of his illness and the rationale of treatment, he cannot be expected to follow through on the treatment plan the doctor recommends. However, the patient responds favorably when the doctor explains arthritis and its natural course. He receives positive support when the doctor tells him how anti-inflammatory drugs, physical and occupational therapy measures, and modern reconstructive joint surgery can help him. But he becomes depressed and suspicious when the doctor gives him superficial information or when he can't understand what the doctor is saying.

Ideally, a physician should: 1) spend sufficient time to give his patients a thorough explanation of the disease, the probable outcome and the reasons for the treatment measures prescribed, and 2) put these medical facts into layman's language which the patient can understand. Knowing what to expect relieves some of the anxiety the patient has about his illness. Knowing what to do about it brightens the patient's outlook and favorably influences the outcome. The physician and patient must be able to talk about both the physical and psychological aspects of arthritis. If the doctor does not have time to inform and to educate his patients personally during the office visit, he can use some of the excellent medically approved booklets and films which are now available to improve the patient's understanding.

The sensitive physician will make every effort to treat the "whole" patient, recognizing clues which reveal a change in the patient's mood and attitudes. The doctor can give the patient a sense of security and provide encouragement and reassurance. The physician's attitude toward the patient helps to determine what the patient's attitude toward his condition will be, and the physician thus plays a key role in the patient's adjustment to and acceptance of his disease.

Let's move on to the relationship between the patient and other health care personnel. What can they do to help the arthritis patient?

The contributions of the public health or visiting nurse can be valuable to both the physician and the patient. The patient may tell medical and personal problems to the nurse which he may conceal from the doctor. The nurse may be able to establish a rapport which allows the patient to feel secure enough to communicate freely. For example, the patient may tell the doctor he is taking the prescribed medication, yet tell the nurse, "I don't take my medicine because I'm afraid of the side effects," or "It doesn't help me anyway." The nurse can check up on how the patient is following the prescribed medical regimen, thus helping both the patient and doctor to follow through on the treatment program.

125

Communicating with Your Professional Health Worker

A home visit can reveal not only how the patient functions in everyday situations, but how his family and home living arrangements may affect his ability to follow the home program the physician has recommended. The nurse can be a link between the doctor and his patient, performing important functions such as 1) helping the patient and family to accept the illness, 2) providing continuing education on various aspects of arthritis, and 3) supplying the doctor with additional information he needs to treat the patient properly.

Physical therapy is often prescribed to help maintain or increase mobility. The patient's first contact with a physical therapist may be when he is taken to the hospital's physical therapy department once or twice a day for treatment. At this time, a physical therapist, following the doctor's orders, will apply the necessary treatments and give instructions for the specific exercises to be performed. The therapist's knowledge and experience in working with arthritis and other chronic musculoskeletal conditions enable him or her to assess the patient's condition, and to be helpful in offering suggestions of ways to more easily accomplish functional and daily living tasks. In working closely with the patient for long periods of time, the therapist has an opportunity to establish a friendly, confident, and secure relationship with him. The therapist, like the visiting nurse, can convey needed information between the physician and patient.

The ambulatory arthritic who is not hospitalized may receive physical therapy through an out-patient clinic. In other instances, the therapist may visit the home to supervise the physical therapy program. There he or she may be able to suggest ways the family members can help the patient cope with any limitations he may have, encourage the family to become involved in the patient's home program, and give helpful suggestions for activities which may motivate the patient to try harder.

In this brief discussion we have not mentioned the medical social worker, occupational therapist, or phychologist. This in no way means that their services are of less value than the others discussed. Each health care worker has much to offer the patient. In addition to bringing a different professional skill to bear on the treatment problems, each can offer invaluable support. As an individual member of the larger medical care team, each professional worker has the responsibility of effective communication with his patient, and of sharing information with other members of the team.

Now that we have outlined the ideal relationship between you, the patient, and the physician, the nurse, and other health care personnel, let's look at your role as a patient. Keep in mind that the goal of both the patient and the medical team is to provide the best possible care to the patient. The patient's effort represents at least half of the treatment program in all chronic disease. With so much depending on you, just what are your responsibilities?

First, you must not ignore the warning signs and symptoms of illness. Carefully select a qualified physician with whom you can openly discuss your condition, then follow his instructions faithfully. You will feel less anxiety if you understand the nature of your illness and the reasons for the treatment program you must follow, so do not hesitate to ask for the information you need. Likewise, you must be open and honest when you communicate with any member of your medical care team. Give realistic data so that accurate assessments can be made. If you have a reaction to medication, increased and prolonged pain following exercise, problems arising from a home program, or any other problems concerning your treatment, these should be reported to your doctor or other health worker.

If you feel you cannot communicate with your health worker, you should approach him with an honest explanation of your dissatisfaction. He may be totally unaware of your feelings. Together, misunderstandings may be resolved. The physician or other health care professional who is doing his best is entitled to know your reasons for lack of confidence before you decide to make a change.

You will do yourself a favor by ignoring the false claims of secret cures, home remedies, and quack treatments and gadgets. Deviation from a medically sound program indicates your lack of confidence in the professionals who are trying to help you manage your arthritis. If you have faith in your professional health care team, you will try to follow the treatment program they have recommended. Your contribution will be that of self-motivation and the determination to stick to the prescribed treatment as long as necessary.

CHAPTER ELEVEN

Psychosocial and Sexual Aspects of Illness

In every illness, there is an interaction between the body and the mind. In order for any treatment to be truly beneficial, the total patient must be considered. Sophisticated machines and new medicines and surgical techniques are making possible improvements in the treatment of many illnesses which not too long ago were considered untreatable. But we also realize that understanding, accepting, and learning to live with illness may be as important to the patient's well-being as dramatic medical advances. Social, cultural, emotional, and personality differences affect the way each one of us responds to the world around us, and these factors in turn will affect how we respond to illness.

One of the most stressful events in anyone's life is learning that he has a chronic illness. Finding out that you have arthritis is a shock. We immediately have visions of being crippled or even bedridden. We fear loss of income, loss of attractiveness, and being a burden on others. Assuming a dependent role may be necessary, and many of us find this very difficult indeed. Most of us have been so geared to "producing" all of our lives that slowing down, working out an easier, less physically and emotionally demanding routine can lead us to feel less adequate than before the illness struck. We may become depressed, fearful, anxious, and angry as a result of learning that we have arthritis. Many of our initial reactions are due to a lack of understanding about the natural course of arthritis. But we now know that sensible combinations of rest, exercise, and medication as prescribed by our physician can help us to lead an active life, and understanding the basic facts about arthritis can set our mind at ease, also.

Pain is often the symptom of arthritis that leads us to seek medical treatment. In addition to obtaining some relief from pain, we need reassurance that we probably won't have to drastically change our lifestyle. We also need to know that our feelings are "normal" and acceptable. Denial or repression of our feelings can lead to tension, both mental and physical. Physical tension can be manifested in an inability to relax, which can develop into a vicious cycle of more and more pain and muscle tightness. Mental tension can cause inability to concentrate, anxiety, and erratic behavior. This constant tension is unproductive, so to counteract it we need to develop sensible ways of facing and dealing with our feelings.

At this point, you may say that it's easier to *talk* about doing something about our feelings than to actually *do* it. But by gaining some insight into what happens to us psychologically when we are ill, we can find ways to avoid letting our feelings upset us unduly. We now want to examine how a person with a chronic illness such as arthritis may feel about himself and the people and world around him.

First of all, let's look at how this person feels about himself. As we said, he may feel inadequate or unable to cope with life. It is very difficult to see ourselves realistically when we are feeling well. It is even more difficult to see ourselves as we really are when we are ill. Part of feeling adequate as a person involves how we feel about our bodies. "Body image" is a name given to the concept of each person's mental picture of his own body. This concept is a dynamic one; it changes in response to what the person perceives is happening to his body. Each person develops a perception of his body through sensory experiences which begin as an infant and continue throughout his entire life. The sum of all these perceptions, which includes the attitudes of his family and friends, contribute to forming a body image.

Body image disturbances can occur when our feelings about our body are unrealistic. For example, we may view minor cosmetic defects as major deformities and alter our behavior accordingly. Or we may believe that we are physically stronger than we really are, and may deny any disabilities we have and attempt to do things beyond our strength. Or the opposite may happen: we may come to believe that we are severely afflicted when such is not the case, and we may not want to go out or do anything at all. The use of prostheses or devices such as braces, walkers, and crutches also can reinforce our feelings of inadequacy and lead to a distorted body image. If we cannot make a realistic assessment of our physical condition, an assess-

Psychosocial and Sexual Aspects of Illness

ment by a trained professional may be in order. Knowing what our limitations and strengths are is essential if we are to accept and learn to live with any chronic illness. Since an accurate, positive body image is so important, we must obtain feedback from others continually so that we can have realistic expectations of ourselves.

Another common problem among people with a chronic illness is loss of self-esteem. Self-esteem is a term meaning self-respect or satisfaction with oneself. Illness often forces us to turn inward, and as a result we may dwell upon our problems excessively. Especially if our mobility is impaired, we feel that we can do very little about even small problems and so we lose any incentive to try to come to grips with our illness. We may despair at accomplishing even necessary daily living tasks. Such despair leads to depression and loss of self-esteem. It is important to combat self-defeating attitudes by setting priorities as to what is most important to us and eliminating unnecessary tasks whenever possible. This is called energy conservation and can apply to mental tasks as well as physical ones. It really is useless to worry about things we can do nothing about; instead, we should try to use our energy in productive ways. If we can visualize that we have only a limited number of units of energy to spend each day, we may become more thrifty in our use of them. The feeling of accomplishment that results can help raise our level of self-esteem.

We do not live in isolation; being members of a social group, a family, and a community, we come into contact with many other persons in the course of our daily lives. No one can be completely self-sufficient, although some persons see this as a worthy goal. It can cause us considerable mental anguish to know that we cannot function on our own, as we have become accustomed to doing. It is not wise to allow others to do so much for us that we feel useless and suffer from lack of exercise and needed activity. But we must learn to ask for and accept help when we really need it, without guilt. If we cannot allow others to show concern for us, we not only make them feel unwanted, we deny them an opportunity to satisfy their need to share with us. This can drive them away from us just when we need them most. False pride can be very destructive to a relationship, and we should guard against it.

Over-protectiveness of family and friends, though well meant, can harm the chronically ill person more than help him. Family members may feel that the arthritis patient cannot or should not engage in certain activities; they may feel that he should not be burdened by family problems; they may try to conceal information about his condition from him. All these tactics can reinforce the patient's feelings of isolation, inadequacy, and guilt. It can be seen that over-protectiveness can be a form of denial and unwillingness of the family to deal with the reality of illness within the family. If one person cannot accept another person's illness, he may try to compensate by showing over-concern, which can cause the patient undue anxiety and does not help him to cope with his illness. Open and honest communication is essential so that suspicions can be laid to rest and the patient feels that he still has something to contribute to others in the family.

While the family members may be over-protective, in many ways they may fail to provide enough psychological support to the patient. Some people are embarrassed or made uncomfortable by illness of another person, and if such a person cannot express these feelings openly, he may appear to reject the patient. The patient then feels that he is no longer acceptable to others and he may withdraw or pretend not to care how others feel about him. The patient needs to feel that his illness is not a source of shame to others and that his friends and family want to help him participate as well as he possibly can in the family and society. If such support is not forthcoming, resentment may result on both sides. The family may feel that the patient is shirking his responsibilities and the patient may feel that he is unfairly being kept out of the mainstream of life.

Much has been written about each person's need for space and privacy, his need to control his environment, and so forth. As we have seen, for the person with chronic illness these may be alien concepts, because he often has little or no personal space, little of no physical or phychological privacy, and precious little control over his environment. If we cannot function without assistance, ordinary daily functions such as climbing stairs, dressing, bathing, and toileting may become traumatic events. Given our Western cultural inclination toward personal privacy, and having been taught that touching implies intimacy, learning to submit to touching when intimacy is not intended can be quite difficult. Trying to unlearn old responses and learn new ones can cause considerable confusion and embarrassment both on the part of the person needing help and the person giving it. Developing a matter-of-fact approach is essential if we are to avoid unnecessary feelings of shame and anxiety in these situations.

Psychosocial and Sexual Aspects of Illness

Now that we have touched on a few potential problem areas concerning the individual and family, let's look at the person with chronic illness in relation to society. For many of us, our job has implications for our feelings of self-esteem and adequacy as a worthy, productive human being. The need to ask for special treatment on the job because of health problems makes us feel different and we also may find that our employer and fellow employees unthinkingly reinforce these differences by fearing that we will be hurt on the job or cause injury to others through our clumsiness. Although such fears may be unrealistic, they are rooted in our suspicion of anyone or anything different. These fears can only be overcome by education and experience, and we may find ourselves in the position of proving that we can function adequately on the job, while also helping others to learn to accept our differences.

The person with a chronic illness may suffer from loss of social status for many reasons, including his inability to participate in community and social affairs, lower income, or even unemployment. This can be a source of worry not only to the person upon whom others are financially dependent, but to anyone who is active in civic and community affairs. The financial hardship imposed by any long-term illness had been well documented. The psychological hardship, while just as critical, is often not talked about. The fewer outlets we have such as work, social and civic activities, and so on, the more time we are forced to spend alone or with only those closest to us. This enforced isolation can cause friction and, again, loss of self-esteem. We all need to feel that we can contribute to society as well as to family life, and being deprived of such

135

opportunities can lead to depression. Although feelings of inadequacy, anxiety, and depression may be only transient, professional help may be indicated if they become our constant companions.

At this point we want to look at another aspect of the total person: sexuality. "Sexuality" is a difficult word or concept to define, but we are using it here in the sense of "the quality or state of being sexual." Our sense of being sexual involves how we feel about ourselves as individuals, as members of a family, and in relation to society.

How we feel about ourselves as sexual beings is influenced by our early experiences, by our relationships with family members and friends, and by our societal and cultural norms. Our individual sexuality is seen in many things we do unconsciously, such as relating differently to men than to women and even in the way we perform daily grooming tasks. Since sexuality is so pervasive, it can be a source of extreme concern when we are not well. And if we are fortunate enough to have a close, loving sexual relationship with someone, we may worry that our illness will interfere with this closeness.

Cultural and societal norms have dictated that masculinity should be exhibited by ability to engage in vigorous physical activity and refusal to acknowledge physical discomfort. This can be devastating to the man with arthritis who is in pain and must curtail some of his activities. One common reaction is denial of physical limitations, with the result that more damage can be incurred by his insisting on doing things beyond his strength. On the other hand, the man with arthritis may suffer loss of libido or sex drive or he may fear that he is unable to perform satisfactorily, and so becomes passive regarding sex. He may then be rejected because he no longer is fulfilling his accustomed "masculine" role of the aggressive, assertive male.

Some women have been conditioned to see themselves as passive and very sensitive in the area of sexual relations. Such a woman may, when she has arthritis, lose all initiative and interest in sex because she feels it is inappropriate for someone in her condition. There may also be a very real fear of being hurt. As a result, her mate feels frustrated and rejected and the relationship may deteriorate. Unfortunately, chronic illness tends to intensify existing problems and may create new ones. The successful resolution of these problems depends on open communication, working to change old habits and ways of relating to one another, and rebuilding the relationship so that each person's needs are met. We need to break down the stereotypes of the strong, dominant male and the silent, passive woman and allow each partner to function within a range of behavior comfortable for him or her.

Some physical problems in sexual functioning can be helped by surgery, especially if these problems are due to deformities which restrict use of certain positions in intercouse. Unrealistic expectations regarding such surgery can be avoided by frank discussion with the orthopedic surgeon or psychological counseling before undertaking the procedure.

One last topic we want to touch on is that of potential side effects of medications on behavior and sexual function. As we know, side effects may occur with some medications used in arthritis management, such as cortisone. These side effects are usually acceptable when weighed against the benefits. However, since medications may affect one person somewhat differently than another person, *behavior* changes may also occur as a result of the medication rather than the illness per se. Muscle relaxants and tranquilizers in particular can depress both physical and psychological ability to function, and if we are unaware of this we can become anxious. We want to stress that any significant behavior changes should be discussed with your health care professional so that an evaluation as to its cause can be undertaken.

One other effect of the need to take medication over an extended period of time is that it may reinforce the image of illness. It has been shown that some persons discontinue medication prematurely, against the physician's directions, because they cannot bear to think of themselves as ill. Particularly in arthritis, a regular regimen of medication can be crucial, and such feelings must be overcome. Some of us may also fear addiction, but the probability of this happening is remote when medications are taken under the direction of a competent physician.

There is no magic cure for the psychological problems that may accompany a chronic illness. As in treatment of your physical condition, patience, knowledge, and healthful practices will go far in helping you to accept and live with your arthritis.

CHAPTER TWELVE

Quackery

No discussion of arthritis treatment would be complete without mentioning the many kinds of quackery currently being perpetrated on arthritis sufferers. The number of fraudulent treatments available are about equal to the number of legitimate ones. Over $485 million a year is spent by arthritis victims in the United States on unproven or worthless forms of arthritis treatment. In this chapter we want to mention some of the more common forms of quackery and give you some guidelines for spotting it.

As we have often said, there is no cure for arthritis. The fact that there is no cure doesn't mean that there are no effective treatments for arthritis, however, and we have told you in other chapters about these accepted and effective treatments.

It is very difficult to prove or disprove the value of many arthritis treatments, for a variety of reasons: first of all, arthritis has a pattern of temporary remission, or disappearance of symptoms, alternating with periods of flare-up. Use of a new treatment may just happen to coincide with a remission, and the patient then mistakenly attributes his apparent improvement to his use of the new remedy. Another difficulty in assessing effectiveness of arthritis treatment is that there is a psychological effect which accompanies *any* treatment, whether good, bad, or indifferent. Just taking action, doing something, puts the patient in a more positive and receptive frame of mind, and this can influence his feelings about whether the treatment is helping him or not. The third factor is the patient's attachment, or lack of it, to the person or physician who is recommending the particular treatment. Because it is human nature to try to please those we care for, a patient is more likely to report favorable results from treatment recommended by someone he likes or has a reason to want to please.

Having given some reasons that accurate assessment of treatments is difficult, let's now discuss some of the unproven, worthless, and dangerous treatments for arthritis.

DIET, VITAMINS, FOLK REMEDIES.

Many medications have their base in folk medicine. Some of these medications, such as digitalis and colchicine, have proven to be valuable. The idea behind the use of folk remedies is that "what is natural is good for you." This idea is especially appealing in today's anti-pollution, back-to-basics culture. But let's examine some of these remedies. For example, apple cider vinegar has been recommended because the acid it contains supposedly helps digest food and it makes body tissue more tender, thus reducing stiffness. There is no scientific evidence for this. Similarly, honey has been touted as a cure-all and most especially as a "purifier" and "joint lubricant." While honey is pleasant tasting and a source high in carbohydrates, its medicinal benefits in arthritis have not been proven. Special diets of many kinds have been promoted, including vitamin regimens which have been "specially formulated" for arthritis. None of these has proven effective; however, if a person is lacking in certain important nutrients and vitamin supplements or a well-balanced diet restores the needed nutrients, he naturally will feel better. It should be noted that some vitamins can be toxic in high dosages. But none of these diets or vitamins can cure arthritis.

COPPER BRACELETS.

There is no evidence that abnormal copper metabolism is a characteristic of any form of arthritis. Neither is there evidence that touching any metal to the skin causes changes in the body. Folklore has it that wearing copper removes electricity from the body, and that the wearing of shoes should be avoided because it prevents release of body electricity into the ground. These theories are scientifically unproven. We all have seen ads for copper bracelets which talk of "vibrations" and "energy fields." One study claims that wearing copper causes "waves" in the area where it touches the skin. None of these claims has been proven.

Quackery

MEXICAN CLINICS.

The so-called "Mexican treatment" has gained notoriety over the past ten years or so. A number of clinics exist in towns just across the border in Mexico. These clinics sell medications which are supposedly curative and not available in the United States. These "cures" have turned out to be cortisone or DMSO, which is a chemical of suspected high toxicity which has not been approved for use in the United States. The high doses given may make the patient feel great for a while, but he then suffers when the treatment wears off and must return for another treatment. Use of any powerful medication without close medical supervision is dangerous.

VACCINES.

About a year ago the *National Enquirer* ran an article citing the claims of a California physician who said that he had developed a vaccine treatment which had ended the pain and stiffness of arthritis in over 500 patients. Supposedly, the treatment worked equally well for RA and osteoarthritis. The Arthritis Foundation made many attempts to obtain information about the vaccine treatment, and investigators from the foundation were not shown any scientific evidence to support any claims that the treatment was effective in either RA or osteoarthritis.

Quackery

HORMONE THERAPY.

The "hormone therapy" which surfaces periodically consists of injecting sex hormones into arthritis patients. This therapy may help reconstruct bone but does nothing else for the joints themselves. Osteoporosis is a condition which involves decreased density of the bones, leading to susceptibility to breakage even in the absence of trauma to the bone, and it occurs sometimes in women past the age of menopause. Osteoporosis is not a form of arthritis, and while hormones may, as we said, help reconstruct bone, they are not effective in treating arthritis. The *National Enquirer* article referred to above claimed hormone therapy to be a cure for arthritis. The Arthritis Foundation investigated and found that the researcher himself said that the article did not properly reflect his research report and that it was exaggerated and sensationalized. So this so-called "cure" has not been confirmed. What *has* been established is that high doses of estrogen, a sex hormone, are dangerous, especially to women over 40. So this treatment should not be looked upon as an arthritis cure until more tests and research are conducted.

ACUPUNCTURE.

While there is some evidence that acupuncture may reduce pain briefly, there has never been any proof that it changes the course of arthritis or any other disease. Some acupuncture practitioners induce some form of hypnotic state in their patients so that at the time they believe themselves to be cured. Acupuncture may be an effective short-term aid to help control pain, but it has not been proven to help arthritis medically.

URANIUM MINES.

It has never been shown that uranium mines are helpful in treating the 3 A's: arthritis, allergy, or asthma, for which sitting in an uranium mine has been claimed to be curative.

To sum up, let us state that a well-balanced diet is important to everyone, sick or well. If you enjoy a particular food in moderation or a particular diet and it isn't harmful, it's probably safe to indulge yourself. And copper bracelets can be very attractive, so if you feel yours adds something to your appearance, go ahead and wear it. But some of the supposed arthritis cures are really dangerous, as we have pointed out, and should, of course, be avoided.

How do you spot someone peddling quackery? Let us quote from the Arthritis Foundation:

1. He may offer a "special" or "secret" formula or device for "curing" arthritis.
2. He advertises. He uses "case histories" and testimonials from satisfied "patients."
3. He may promise (or imply) a quick or easy cure.
4. He may claim to know the cause of arthritis and talk about "cleansing" your body of "poisons" and "pepping up" your health. He may say surgery, x-rays, and drugs prescribed by a phyician are unnecessary.

5. He may accuse the "medical establishment" of deliberately thwarting progress, or of persecuting him . . . but he doesn't let his method be tested in tried and proved ways.

Check with your doctor or the Arthritis Foundation or other recognized authority before trying any new treatment for arthritis. Your health is too valuable to risk losing or damaging it.

CHAPTER THIRTEEN

Therapeutic Recreation for Persons with Arthritis

The concept of therapeutic recreation and its definition as meaningful, goal-directed activity have come about as a result of several factors. One of these is the over-abundance of leisure time that more and more persons now have, and the other is the need of persons with physically disabling conditions for activities and exercises which have the express purpose of helping them to minimize or overcome their functional limitations. Such persons need the low-cost alternatives to television, cards, and passive games that can be provided by a well-thought-out individual or group program of therapeutic recreation.

The goals of therapeutic recreation are to: 1) restore self-care, 2) promote and maintain normal living activities, and 3) provide social and psychological benefits to the participants. It goes without saying that individual capacities and interests must be a major consideration when planning any recreation program. Another consideration is to be certain that participation is voluntary— no one wants to feel that he is being forced to do something he really doesn't want to do! Fortunately, many of our daily interests and hobbies can provide a basis for each one of us to develop a recreation program tailored to our individual interests and needs.

Some of us may hesitate to join in recreational activities because we have grown up in a society centered around the "work ethic." In such an environment, we become prejudiced against anything regarded as "play" and may actually feel guilty about taking time for ourselves just for the sheer enjoyment of it. Therapeutic recreation can provide the goal for our having fun—we can indulge in some enjoyable activity while helping exercise the parts of our bodies that need special attention!

Unfortunately, recreation of any kind holds a low priority not only in many persons' minds, but in the eyes of many persons in city governments, community agencies, and health care facilities. Such persons are often in a position to provide some funds and personnel for programs for those with special needs, but don't want to be accused of spending resources on "frivolous" programs. In larger cities, community recreation programs sometimes offer a wide range of activities for persons of various interests, abilities, and ages. While some smaller communities may have recreation facilities and programs, others may not. This is especially true of rural areas, where most activities are centered around the family, church, and clubs. In such cases, programs may still be developed for those with special needs if someone will take the lead in suggesting to the local minister or club president that such a service project would fill a need and also be a fulfilling activity for the members of the club or congregation.

Historically, the concept of therapeutic recreation goes back to Greek times. It was a dynamic concept which promoted development of the body and correction of any deficiencies in functioning. The Romans further refined the idea, and Galen, a physician who practiced in the second century A.D., mentioned the highly organized, elaborate structure of public games, contests, and other activities designed to help the citizens realize their potential as well-rounded individuals. Today, the concept fits in nicely with our modern idea of health as one's capacity for coping with or adapting effectively to all the physical, emotional, social, intellectual, and economic demands of his environment. Through therapeutic recreation, we have an opportunity for physical activity, emotional release, social involvement, and creative expression. All of these contribute to maintaining good health.

Therapeutic recreation for the person with arthritis can be an extension of exercises performed specifically for maintaining and increasing joint range of motion and muscle strength. We often tend to overlook the very real benefits to our bodies to be gained from our hobbies and daily activities. For example, finger painting, making collages, and even gardening can help maintain finger dexterity, and other hobbies can exercise other parts of

148

the body. A recreational activity usually can be found that will help exercise a particular part of the body and so combine fun with therapy. While it would be impossible to list all such activities, we will attempt to suggest a few which are especially applicable to the person with arthritis.

Those of us who like to feel that we are contributing to the welfare of others by working on projects that directly benefit others in need will find satisfaction in making toys for bazaars, beanbags for day care centers, or addressing and stuffing envelopes for charities. All these provide good exercise for the hands.

The less severely involved arthritic who enjoys music and dancing might consider joining a square dancing group. If done smoothly, without stomping or other jerky movements which can aggravate affected joints, square dancing can provide good exercise as well as enjoyable social contact. And, of course, ballroom dancing, which is again popular, is a means of self-expression and promotes good circulation and coordination.

Music offers the opportunity for individual expression and also affords the person with arthritis another opportunity to exercise the parts of his body that need attention. Playing a keyboard instrument such as the organ, piano, or xylophone exercises the upper torso, hands, and shoulders. Using the pedals can help maintain flexibility in the legs and feet. The woodwind and stringed instruments such as the guitar and banjo help exercise the muscles of the fingers and wrists. Singing and playing woodwind instruments can relax and strengthen the muscles of the face, throat, and chest, and improve

149

breathing. Lack of real musical talent need not deter us—everyone can play some instrument or hum or sing along!

A love of flowers or birds can be developed into a stimulating activity which combines walking with the pleasure of identifying different species. Armed with a pocket book which lists characteristics of each species and location where found, along with a picture in most cases, we can even become experts. This can also lead to very interesting discussions with other persons with similar interests.

Swimming as therapy is covered elsewhere in this book, so it will not be discussed in this section. It should be stressed, however, that any type of exercise performed in the water is especially helpful to the arthritic because of the buoyancy the water provides.

Women's magazines and special arts and crafts publications are good sources for low-cost, interesting, and useful handicraft projects. Many require a minimum of tools and some even re-cycle materials. The sense of accomplishment that comes with creating a decoration for the home or gift gives our spirits a lift, while the actual work that goes into making the item may provide valuable exercise.

Golf and bowling have become popular recreational activities in this country which offer exercise, social contact, and a feeling of pride in a well-played game to even the relatively unskilled participant. A word of caution may be in order, however, for the person with arthritis who enjoys these sports. Although trial-and-error experimentation will permit you to learn just what you can and cannot tolerate, you can avoid painful strains by remembering and applying the energy-saving and joint-protection principles discussed elsewhere in this book. When bowling, you must be certain that the weight of the ball and the necessary arm swing do not place undue strain upon any joints. Likewise, the golfer should take care not to strain any joints with which he has experienced problems. Using a motorized golf cart will avoid the need to carry a heavy golf bag or to pull a wheeled caddy. The latter practice can place the person pulling the caddy in some very awkward positions which can aggravate arthritic problems in the shoulders, arms, and back. In any sport, you must learn your limitations and adjust your play accordingly so as not to place additional stress upon the parts of your body which have been weakened.

The outdoors-loving person with arthritis will find that he still can enjoy many activities. So long as you wear properly fitted footgear, do not carry a heavily loaded backpack which places undue strain on the back, shoulders, hips, and legs, and do not become excessively fatigued, you can continue to hike in easy terrain. Of course, serious mountain-climbing is only for the most hardy, and will usually be beyond the ability of anyone with more than "a touch" of arthritis. You should, as always, be guided by feedback from your body.

The benefits of walking cannot be over-emphasized. A walking program involves little expense beyond investment in some proper footgear (no high heels, please!) and comfortable clothing. Walking can be enjoyed at all times of the year with the exception of days when extreme weather conditions make footing treacherous or the walker uncomfortably warm or cold. It not only builds up the legs, thus increasing capacity in the circulatory and respiratory systems, but it also can improve coordination and overall fitness. Some experimentation will help you find the route, distance, and speed best suited to your abilities. *Regularity* is the key to any exercise program, so, if possible, walk at the same time or times each day. If your endurance, strength, or time are limited, you may find it easier to walk for even five or ten minutes several times a day. So much the better if you can persuade a friend to join you, because then you can share experiences along the way and both of you will enjoy walking much more!

Interest in Eastern philosophy and exercise systems has made "yoga" a household word in the last few years. Many persons now perform yoga while watching one of the popular television programs where attractive ladies demonstrate the positions and provide encouragement, or participate in yoga classes sponsored by the YMCA or other community recreation agencies. Some of the easier positions can help maintain joint range of motion and flexibility, but, again, a word of caution to the arthritic: the more strenuous positions should be avoided because of the potential strain they place upon body parts that may in the arthritic have become relatively immobile or are painful. As with any exercise, pain that lasts more than an hour or so is a sign that the exercise should probably be discontinued.

Another system of body positions and gentle exercises called Tai Chi can be of help in maintaining flexibility while not placing excessive strain on organs and joints that may not be functioning at maximum capacity. Qualified instructors for many of these Eastern disciplines can now be found in many communities, and some offer a trial lesson so that you can determine if the exercises are compatible with your physical limitations.

Your doctor should be consulted before you decide to begin any strenuous or new program. If he approves, start slowly and build capacity gradually. A "slow and easy" approach will pay off in avoiding soreness, further damage, and disappointment. You will then truly benefit from the therapeutic recreation program you have become involved in.

CHAPTER FOURTEEN

Pool Exercise Program

A regular pool exercise program performed in a swimming pool has many benefits for the person with arthritis. Pool exercise can provide the arthritic with a safe, non-strenuous recreational opportunity that generally will not contribute to further joint destruction. Many arthritics are exhilarated to find that water presents a medium in which much more movement can be obtained than on land. Frequently, longer periods of exercise can be tolerated so that muscle strength and joint range of motion are gained and maintained with greater ease.

Many parts of the body which are commonly affected by arthritis can be successfully exercised in the pool. For example, arthritics with hip or knee joint involvement frequently discover that walking in chest-deep water is easier and less painful than on land. Exercising an affected shoulder in the pool can also be less painful because of the cushioning support given to the arm by the water. Furthermore, swimming and appropriate pool exercises are excellent conditioning techniques for those with semi-acute and chronic low back pain due to arthritis of the spine. For examples of specific exercises and strokes recommended, refer to the exercise section at the end of this chapter.

Water possesses two properties which make its use ideal as an exercise medium: buoyancy and mass. First, movement is easier in water because of its buoyancy. If the body part is moved slowly underwater, the water acts as an assist or support to that movement. Such assistance effectively reduces the weight of the body part and thereby minimizes the stress placed on the joint when motion is initiated. With reduced stress, the joint is able to move through a greater range of motion with significantly less pain. If you have limitation in range of motion as well as strength, we recommend that the goals of your pool exercise program be initially to increase your range of motion, and later to increase strength.

Walking activities can be easily practiced in a pool. The water reduces the total weight of the body, thus minimizing the many pounds of pressure placed on the hip, knee, and ankle joints during gait maneuvers. On days when a weight-bearing joint is too painful on land, a good walk can still be accomplished without increased pain in the pool. Walking exercises in the water can help improve standing posture and sometimes help develop a limp-free gait.

Pool exercise may be additionally beneficial in promoting relaxation. The heat of the water, increased activity, and feeling of weightlessness combine to allow increased relaxation of the musculature with an overall reduction of tension level. Such exercise and recreation help relieve the pent-up feelings of anger and anxiety which often accompany chronic illness.

Deep breathing is facilitated by underwater exercise. The pressure of the water resists exhalation efforts and consequently strengthens the lower chest wall musculature. Slow and deep breathing exercises practiced in chest-deep water can help improve posture as well as expand the capacity of the rib cage.

Other benefits from exercising in a pool include increased circulation from increased activity, possible reduction of swelling of the extremeties, and improved coordination. Of the greatest benefit, however, is the pure recreational pleasure to be gained from participating in the sport and skills of aquatics. Combining a pool exercise program with family recreation or socializing with a group of friends who also enjoy the water can make needed exercise fun and inviting.

A pool exercise program can be performed standing at various depths of water, sitting in shallower areas, or may incorporate normal swimming maneuvers for those who have had some previous swimming experience. Inflatable devices for supporting the body in the water while allowing freedom of arm and leg movements can be used by those who cannot swim.

Many apartment complexes, condominiums, and retirement centers offer swimming pool facilities for their residents. YMCA's and other public recreation centers often reserve certain time periods for swimming for handicapped persons and senior citizens. Some facilities have made special provisions for the swimmer with limited mobility so that there is easy and safe access to the pool and dressing rooms. Some pools have a hydraulic lift which is especially useful for the severely involved arthritic who cannot use steps easily.

Although pool water temperature cannot be regulated by each individual user, the most comfortable temperature range for the arthritic is between 88° and 96° F. Although application of ice can be very helpful in relieving joint pain, water that is too cold not only feels unpleasant on the body and may cause chilling, but it can increase joint pain. Also, the air above the pool should be comfortably warm and draft-free to prevent chilling when leaving the pool.

Your swimsuit should be as lightweight as possible and not restrict your freedom of movement. Materials such as denim and terrycloth absorb the water, becoming very heavy and unsuitable as you leave the pool and attempt to remove the garment. A nylon tank suit is the best type of suit for a woman, as it is lightweight, non-restricting, and dries quickly. Towels and wrap-up apparel should be immediately handy upon leaving the pool in order to prevent chilling.

The duration of the exercise session will depend upon the temperature of the water, how comfortable you feel in an aquatic environment, and the severity of your arthritic condition. The length of the exercise period may vary widely, from about ten minutes to an hour. Shorter time periods are advised for initial sessions, and then the time can gradually be increased.

Any swimmer, and especially the arthritic, should have some way to summon assistance while exercising in the pool. A loud bell or horn can be used to attract attention, or someone can be asked to stay near the pool so that he can summon additional help if needed. If you need assistance to enter or leave the pool, you should be certain that someone is nearby. The easiest access to a pool is by means of wide steps which have a railing nearby at the shallow end of the pool. Handrails or grips are helpful for underwater exercise, but they are not essential.

You may find that life jackets and inflatable headrests help you to obtain good, safe positioning for exercising in the pool. Stools and chairs placed in the shallow area are useful for necessary rest periods and for use while exercising your arms. They should be made of stainless steel and be adequately weighted so that they remain at the bottom of the pool. Lawn chairs, plastic chairs, or metal benches may be substituted, if properly weighted. Remember that chlorine-treated water will deteriorate most materials, especially rubber.

After leaving the pool, you should shower to rinse off any chlorine from the water that remains on your skin. Some arthritics who take certain medications such as Motrin and some of the corticosteroid derivatives may experience skin reactions such as itching, and a rash may develop as a result. The reaction can be minimized by showering immediately after swimming.

The person with arthritis must be cautious to avoid over-activity, strain, and excessive fatigue. Any increase in pain should last no longer than one hour after finishing the activity.

Pool exercise is contraindicated if you have one or more of the following health problems:

1. Fever.
2. Some heart conditions (check with your physician).

3. Some chest diseases (check with your physician).
4. Some kidney conditions (check with your physician).
5. Markedly high blood pressure.
6. Contagious skin diseases.
7. Open wounds.
8. Some allergic conditions (check with your physician).

Armed with knowledge as to your tolerance for activity and a willingness to experiment a bit, you can develop a regular pool exercise program that will not only help you to increase your joint range of motion and strength, but will also be enjoyable, especially if a friend will join you. On the following pages are suggested pool exercises for all parts of the body.

Note: Some of the materials used in preparation of this chapter are from *Therapeutic Pools; Programs and Management* (to be published) by Mary Carpenter, R.P.T.

SUGGESTED POOL EXERCISES

I. Foot and Ankle Exercises
   1. Stand on bottom of the pool in chest-deep water, holding onto the edge for support.
      a. Stand on heels. Relax.
      b. Stand on toes. Relax.
      c. Stand on outer borders of the feet. Relax.
      d. Repeat sequence.
   2. Bob up and down in shoulder-deep water.
   3. Floating on your back or sitting in the pool, rotate both feet at the same time in a circle. Then circle in the opposite direction.

4. Flutter kick. The flutter kick is similar to a normal walking step. While holding the side of the pool with both hands and facing forward, extend the legs in back and let them float. Simply move one leg and then the other as though you were walking. Both hip and knee action are used. Keep the legs relaxed and let the knee lead the kick. The legs should not break the surface of the water. The flutter kick can be done on the back also.

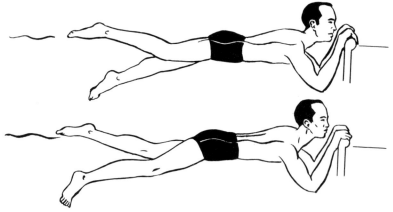

Figure 29.   Flutter kick.

5. Scissors Kick. Start with both legs extended as in walking. Bend the knees and bring legs up toward the chest while separating legs. Bring one leg forward and the other back toward the rear. Then bring both legs together in a rapid movement, straightening them to initial position. Repeat sequence.

160

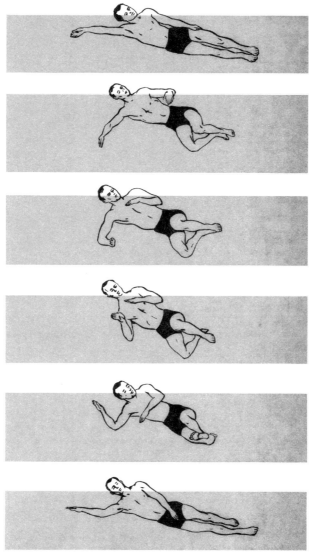

Figure 30. Scissor kick.

Pool Exercise Program

II. Knee Exercises

    1. Standing on the bottom of the pool in waist-deep water and holding onto the edge for support, bend both knees as if to squat; bend as far as possible without pain. Straighten to standing position and repeat.

    2. Bob up and down in chest-deep water, flexing the knees.

    3. Sitting on a stool or the steps of the pool, bend and straighten knee with leg out in front of body. Alternate knees.

    4. Flutter kick.

    5. Scissors kick.

III. Hip Exercises

    1. Standing in shallow water, squat on the bottom of the pool, holding onto the edge for support. Use leg muscles to push into standing position. Repeat.

    2. Standing in the pool in chest-deep water and holding onto the edge for support:

        a. Swing leg forward, keeping the knee straight.

        b. Swing leg backward without bending the upper body forward.

        c. Swing leg out to the side, keeping the knee straight.

    3. Walk sideways in the pool.

    4. Walk backwards in the pool.

    5. Flutter kick.

    6. Scissors kick.

Pool Exercise Program

IV. Shoulder Exercises
1. Bending forward in chest-deep water, swing arm forward and backward in pendular fashion. This exercise may be performed while sitting or standing.
2. In shoulder-deep water, sit or stand with arms outstretched at shoulder height to the sides. Make circles with your arms, starting with small ones and progressing to larger ones.

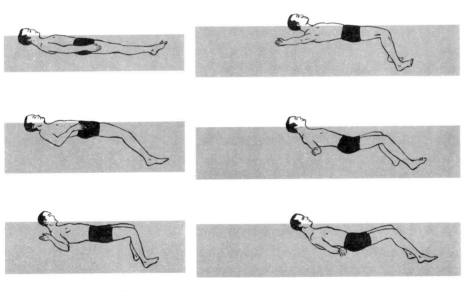

Figure 31. Elementary backstroke.

3. Elementary Backstroke. Float on the back with arms at sides. Bend elbows and bring hands along sides up to armpits. Straighten arms out to sides, even with the shoulders. Push arms down to

163

sides, palms facing body. Arms should be underwater. The frog kick (shown in section on low back exercises) or other kick can be combined with this movement.

4. Finning. Floating on the back, with arms extended down at the sides, draw your hands up along the sides of the body to about hip level. Elbows will be bent but not at right angles to the body. Extend the fingertips outward, then move the hands and arms backward toward the feet. Return to original position and repeat. This movement will be quite natural and will propel you backward in the water.

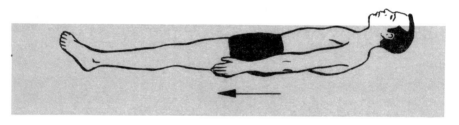

Figure 32. Finning.

5. Sculling. Floating on the back, hold arms at the sides in a relaxed position. Press hands outward with the wrists leading and little fingers slightly up toward the surface of the water. Return the hands toward the body with wrists leading and thumbs slightly upward. Move the hands continuously in this pattern. The pushing out and pulling in will make a figure 8 pattern.

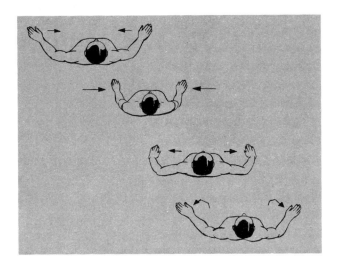

Figure 33. Sculling.

V. Low Back Exercises
  1. Standing in chest-deep water with back against
     the pool wall, slowly bring one knee up toward
     your chest while maintaining pelvic tilt. Pelvic tilt
     is accomplished by tightening abdominal muscles
     and tucking the buttocks under so that the curve
     in the lower back is minimized. Alternate knees.
  2. While sitting in shallow water, bend both knees
     and bring toward chest.
  3. While sitting in shallow water, alternate knees to
     chest.
  4. Walk in the pool on your toes while maintaining a
     pelvic tilt.

165

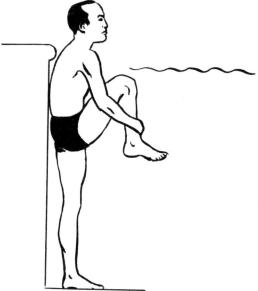

Figure 34. Low back exercises.

5. Walk in the pool in a marching fashion, bringing each knee as high as possible while maintaining pelvic tilt.
6. Elementary backstroke (especially for acute periods).
7. Tread water using various kicks—scissors, bicycle, and frog. The bicycle is an up-and-down movement from hip to toe, as in pedalling a bicycle. The frog kick is performed by bringing the heels together, bending the knees up and out. With ankles bent, spread feet far apart. Straighten legs outward, then bring them together as quickly as possible.

Pool Exercise Program

AVOID STROKES CAUSING EXCESSIVE BACK EXTENSION AND ARCHING SUCH AS THE BREAST STROKE, DOG PADDLE, AND FRONT CRAWL WITH FACE UP OUT OF THE WATER.

CHAPTER FIFTEEN

Exercises

On the following pages your will find the Personal Health Services Home Program exercises. This exercise program has been designed by physical therapists for the arthritis patient who wants to remain mobile and continue to participate in family and social life. There are two aims of the exercise program: 1) to maintain and increase joint range of motion of all parts of the body, and 2) to provide the patient with exercises for specific problem areas. These exercises, in combination with the joint protection principles, hints for performing daily living tasks more easily, and other materials in this book, can help the arthritic to learn to live with, not for, his arthritis.

Instructions for Developing Your Home Exercise Program

In an ideal situation, the arthritic is under the care of a competent physician who has both expertise and experience with rheumatological diseases, and the mutual relationship is such that they can and do communicate well with one another. The patient, from experience and from information given to him by his physician and other health professionals, knows the nature of his own condition and what the future holds in relation to his illness, his limitations in functioning at his job, at home, and within social situations.

Armed with all this information and supported by the professional expertise of this physician and allied health professionals, our "ideal arthritic" can develop a program of home exercises designed to help maintain and increase his joint range of motion. But what about those arthritics who are faced with a less than ideal situation? How can you develop an exercise program that can be conveniently performed at home that will help you remain active and enjoy life more?

On the following pages are groups of exercises designed for specific areas of the body most commonly affected by arthritis. As these exercises are used, it is important to remember the material in the chapter on "Posture, Rest and Exercise." Here is a review of the seven rules for exercise:

Rule 1. You are an individual. Your home exercise program will not be structured exactly like another arthritic's exercise program. Your joint involvement and tolerance to exercise may be very different. Set your own goals realistically and adopt a reasonable exercise program that you can faithfully follow.

Rule 2. Start exercising slowly and carefully. Do each exercise three to five times initially, then gradually increase the repetitions as your tolerance permits. Perform the exercise smoothly. Avoid sudden, jerky, and rapid movements.

Rule 3. Most exercise programs can be performed in two sessions of fifteen to twenty minutes daily. Make these sessions part of your daily routine.

Rule 4. When your illness is acute and you are having a joint "flare-up" you must considerably reduce or cease active exercise to that particular joint. During this time, you may use assisted or isometric exercise. As the joint inflammation and pain subsides, you may gradually resume active exercise to regain strength and endurance.

Rule 5. You may, and probably will, experience increased pain after exercising, especially if you start too vigorously. If discomfort from exercise continues longer than an hour, decrease the amount of exercise.

Rule 6. Don't expect too much too soon! Accept each day as a step nearer to your individual goal.

Rule 7. Start today.

Proceeding cautiously and at a reasonable pace, begin performing the exercises for that part of your body which has been properly diagnosed as arthritic. Complete each exercise to the best of your ability. If you cannot perform an exercise, you may have a friend or family member gently move your arm or leg as the exercise prescribes. Do the exercises twice daily. Then as the days go by, work to increase the number of repetitions, your range of motion, and coordination.

As your exercise program progresses, slowly add recommended exercises for other parts of your body to maintain strength, range of motion, and posture. These maintenance exercises may be done three times a week.

Incorporate your exercise program with your routine

Exercises

HOME EXERCISE PROGRAM

CHART

TO BE USED WHEN LEARNING THE EXERCISES FOR THE
VARIOUS PARTS OF THE BODY

NUMBER OF REPETITIONS

EXERCISE	WEEK 1	WEEK 2	WEEK 3	WEEK 4	WEEK 5
Range of Motion					
Breathing					
Hip					
Knee					
Shoulder					
Arm					
Neck					
Finger					
Wrist					
Hand					
Toe					
Elbow					

daily activities. Arm and hand exercises may be performed during your favorite daytime television program. Hip exercises may be performed while working at a desk or table. You may find that an exercise session before going to bed at night will reduce morning stiffness and pain. Your exercise program should become as automatic as eating, bathing, and all other things we do almost without thinking each day.

Remember to exercise with caution. On days when you don't feel well, exercise less. If you must stop for a few days, start again gradually. Don't try to catch up in a few days. Regularity is the key to any exercise program—it must be continued for the rest of your life, not just performed on the days you feel you have the time or remember to fit in a few. We believe that if you will follow the hints we have given, make use of the information elsewhere in this book, and follow the home exercise program you develop on a regular basis, you will be rewarded by feeling much more fit and be able to perform needed tasks more easily.

JOINT RANGE OF MOTION EXERCISES— LOWER EXTREMITY

I. Hip: Do exercises while standing
   A. Flexion—bending.
   B. Extension—straightening.
   C. Abduction—taking leg away from center of body.
   D. Adduction—bringing leg closer to center of body.

Exercises

E. Rotation—Internal: turn leg in toward center.
External: turn leg out away from center.

F. Circumduction—taking leg in circular motion.

II. Knee
  A. Flexion—bending leg.
  B. Extension—straightening leg.

III. Ankle
  A. Dorsiflexion—bend ankle and point toes toward head.
  B. Plantarflexion—straighten ankle and point toes down toward floor.
  C. Inversion—turning toes in.
  D. Eversion—turning toes out.
  E. Circumduction—moving in a circular motion.

IV. Toes
  A. Flexion—bending all joints so that toes curl under.
  B. Extension—straightening all toes.
  C. Abduction—separating toes.
  D. Adduction—bringing toes together.

JOINT RANGE OF MOTION EXERCISES—
UPPER EXTREMITY

  I. Shoulder
  A. Flexion—lift arm up over head.
  B. Extension—take arm down and backward.
  C. Abduction—take arm away from body.

173

Exercises

    D. Adduction—bring arm in toward body.

    E. Rotation—Internal: turn arm toward body.

          External: turn arm away from body.

    F. Circumduction—move arm in circular motion.

II. Elbow

    A. Flexion—bend elbow toward shoulder with hand facing up.

    B. Extension—straighten elbow and move forearm downward.

    C. Pronation—holding arm at side, turn elbow so that palm of hand faces down.

    D. Supination—holding arm at side, turn elbow so that palm of hand faces up.

III. Wrist

    A. Flexion—bend.

    B. Extension—straighten.

    C. Ulnar deviation—turn wrist toward little finger.

    D. Radial deviation—turn wrist toward thumb.

    E. Circumduction—circular motion of wrist.

IV. Fingers

    A. Flexion—bending all joints.

    B. Extension—straightening all joints.

    C. Abduction—separating fingers.

    D. Adduction—bringing fingers together.

    E. Opposition—bringing thumb to fingers.

    F. Circumduction—moving fingers in a circular motion.

Exercises

BREATHING EXERCISES

Objectives:
1. To develop good posture habits and proper breathing techniques.
2. To discourage fast and shallow breathing and encourage slower and deeper breaths.
3. To stretch chest muscles and expand the rib cage capacity.

Breathing Exercises:
1. Backlying or sitting: Place hands on sides of chest; inhale deeply, pushing your ribs out against your hands. Exhale, blowing excess air out through your mouth.
2. Backlying: Bend knees, keep arms at sides. Raise both arms overhead while inhaling deeply. Hold; exhale slowly as arms are lowered to sides.
3. Backlying: Bend knees, keep soles of feet flat on the floor. Press feet into floor; tighten abdominal muscles; lift head and curl up towards a semi-sitting position, reaching toward your knees with outstretched arms. Exhale as your curl; inhale as you uncurl and relax.
4. Backlying or sitting: Place hands on upper abdomen. Take short, quiet breaths through your mouth (panting), followed by a long hissing expiration. Pressure of hands may be gradually increased during inhalation.
5. Backlying: Breathe out slowly, sinking the chest as

175

much as possible, then the upper abdomen. Place hands on lower margins of the rib cage. Relax the abdomen so that it swells a little and the lower part of the chest expands slightly, while inhaling quickly and silently through the nose. Do *not* raise the chest.

6. Flex arms and slowly rise on toes to maximum height possible. Hold, then slowly lower arms to sides. Inhale deeply while rising on toes and hold. Exhale while lowering arms.

7. Standing: Same as number 6 except take a few steps while standing on toes, still holding breath before release.

8. Forced Exhalation:
   A. Sitting: With arms hanging down toward floor, bend head forward on chest and force *all* air from lungs.
   B. Backlying: Breathe in normally. Exhale *all* air, making a whistle while doing so. This resists the outgoing air, strengthening the bronchial tubes, and more effectively empties the lungs so that air intake is increased.

9. Activities:
   A. Practice deep breathing in fresh air and/or following exercise of a more vigorous nature.
   B. Blow up balloons.
   C. Blow ping-pong balls or cotton balls across a table.
   D. Suck in on a dry straw and blow out.

Exercises

SHOULDER EXERCISES

Standing

    1. Shrug shoulders upward, then pull shoulders down. Relax and repeat.

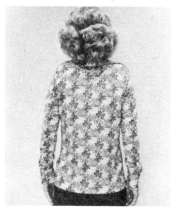 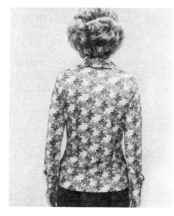

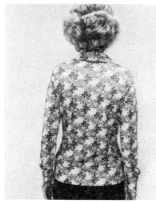

Exercises

2. Pull shoulders forward, then pull shoulders backward. Relax and repeat.
3. Combine upward, forward, downward and backward motions above in a circular motion.
4. Pendulum exercises - Bend at waist, bracing with left arm on a countertop, table, etc. Let right arm hang in a relaxed position.

   a.) Swing arm forward.

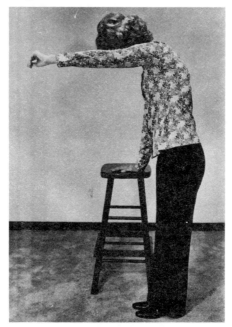

   b.) Swing arm backward.
   c.) Swing arm away from body.
   d.) Swing arm toward body.
   e.) Combine all of the above motions in a circle (clockwise then counterclockwise).

   Repeat with left arm.

5. Bending elbows, place finger tips on shoulders. Rotate elbows in circular fashion - first clockwise then counterclockwise.

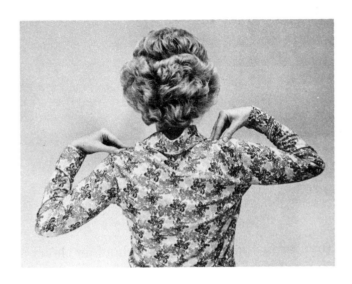

6. Using a cane, broom handle, baton, etc. Grasp cane with both hands and:
   a.) Lift arms up over head.
   b.) Take arms down to sides.
   c.) Swing arms to the right side.
   d.) Swing arms to the left side.
   e.) Lift arms up over head, bend elbows and slide cane *down* back.

Exercises

f.) Hold cane behind you and slide it *up* the back.

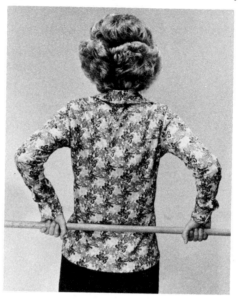

7. Hold arms outstretched at shoulder level. Make circles. Relax and change direction.

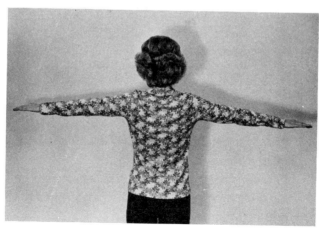

180

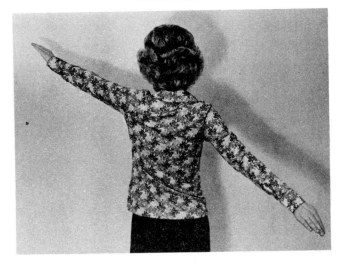

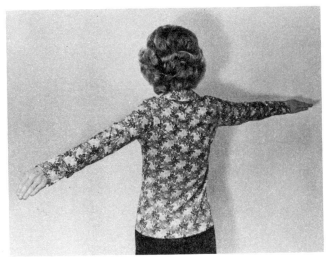

Sitting

The above exercises (1-7) may be done in a sitting position

Backlying
　1.　Lift arms together or alternately over head.

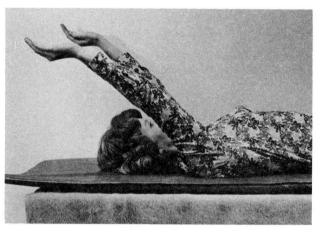

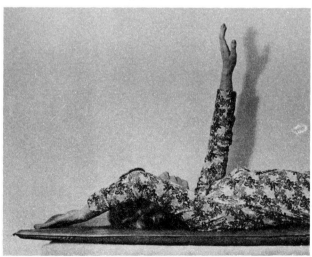

2. Lower arms together or alternately down to sides.
3. Extend arms together or alternately out to sides (away from body).
4. Bring arms together or alternately in to body.
5. With arms out to side at shoulder level and elbows bent, lower hands forward toward bed, then raise them backward.
6. With arms straight at sides, turn arms in and then out. (Palms of hands alternately up then down.)

Facelying with small pillow under abdomen
1. Lift both arms together or alternately from bed or floor. Relax and repeat.

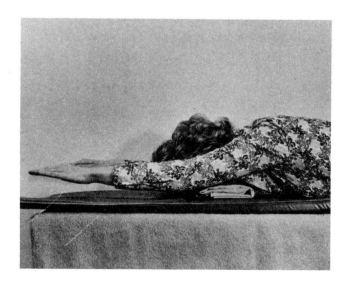

2. Clasp hands behind back, let elbows bend while bringing hands up toward shoulder blades.

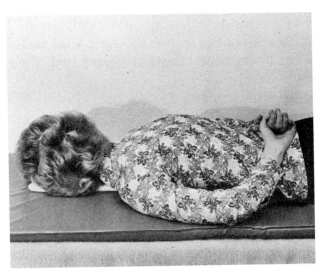

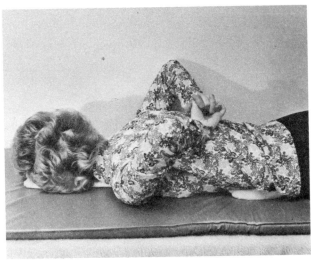

184

3. Clasp hands behind neck and pull elbows up and back.

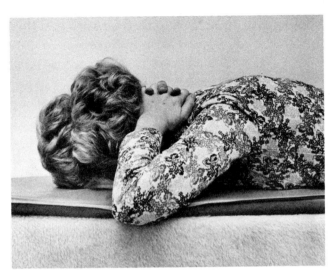

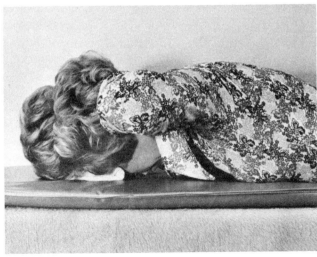

Exercises

4. Extend right arm away from side and even with the shoulder. Keep the arm supported on the bed as far as the elbow. With forearm hanging off the bed and with elbow bent, bring hand forward and then take it backward. Repeat with left arm.

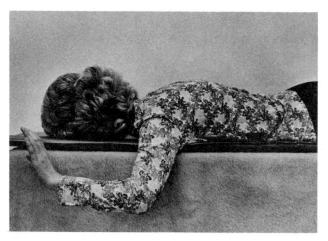

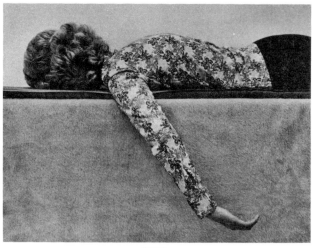

Exercises

ARM EXERCISES

Objective:

The following exercises are given to promote flexibility and strength of the shoulders and arms. They should be performed to the fullest range of motion possible.

1. *Rubber Ball Exercise* - You will need a rubber ball with a rubber string. Begin by simply squeezing the ball to strengthen the grip. Then throw the ball away from body in different directions to encourage greater motion.

2. *Wall Climbing* - With feet well balanced, and toes about 6″ from wall, face the wall and rest your forehead against it. Slowly reach with your arms

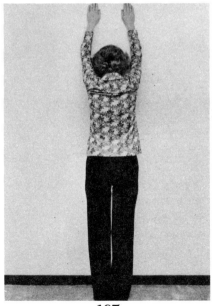

187

along the wall over your head. Try to increase the length of the reach each time.

3. *Rope Exercise* (Improvised Shoulder Wheel) - Use a piece of rope the length of your outstretched arm. Tie it to a doorknob, cabinet or drawer knob, etc. Stand with feet well balanced with side facing the rope. Take the rope in your hand on that side and put the opposite hand on your hip for balance. Without bending your arm or waist and using your shoulder, turn the rope as if turning a jump rope. Do this in both directions and repeat with the opposite arm.

4. *Pulley Exercise* - A swivel pulley with a soft piece of rope knotted or looped at each end inserted through

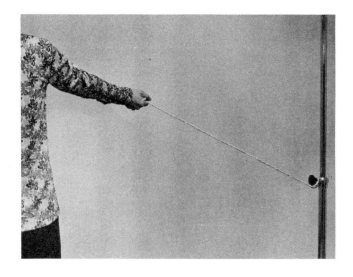

it may be attached to a beam, door frame, etc. Sit or stand underneath the pulley and put the second and third fingers of each hand through loops or knots. Pull down on rope with one hand, taking the opposite arm up. Different directions can be done depending on the position of the pulley attachment and the patient. If you cannot attach a pulley, the rope may be placed over a shower rod, other rods, or a hook attached to a wall or door.

5. *Paper Crumple* - Place a stack (15 sheets) of old newspapers (tabloid size) on the table. Rest forearm on the table with hand on the corner of the pile. Crumple each sheet separately and discard. Repeat the exercise using the opposite arm.

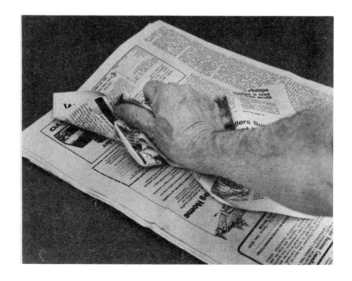

6. *Rod Exercise* - Stand with arms straight in front of you holding a rod (cane, broom handle). With elbows straight, raise the rod over your head. Relax and bend elbows, lowering the rod behind your head. Variation: grasp rod with arms behind you and lift it toward upper back by bending elbows.

FINGER EXERCISES

1. With hand resting on table and palm up:

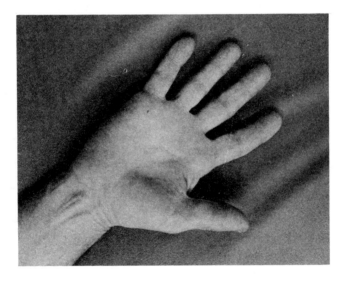

a) Make a tight fist by squeezing. Relax and straighten fingers on table.

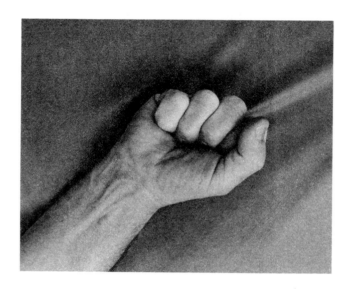

b) Bring tips of fingers to area where they join the hand. Relax and straighten.
c) Bring tips of fingers toward wrist. Relax and straighten.
d) Oppose thumb to each of the other fingers (i.e., touch tip of thumb to the tip of each finger, one at a time).

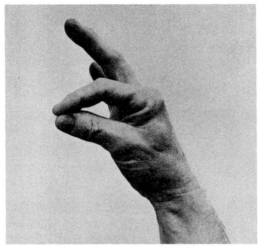

e) Rotate thumb in a circular motion.
f) Separate all the fingers (including thumb).
g) Bring all fingers together.

2. With hand resting on a table and palm down:

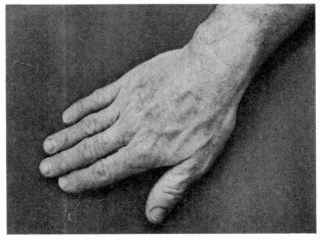

Exercises

a) Separate all fingers.

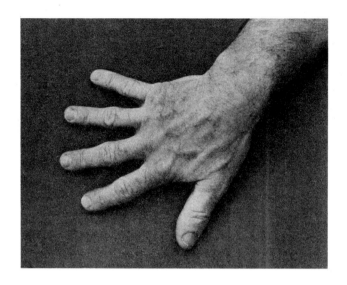

b) Bring all fingers together.

c) Lift all the fingers (including thumb) first separately, then together.

d) With wrist flat on the table, press down and draw fingers into a "clawing" position, then straighten.

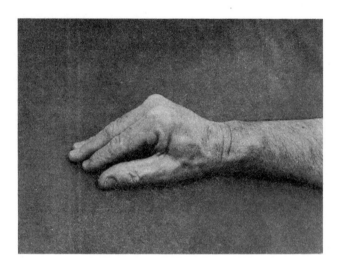

You may use one hand, or the fingers thereof, to assist or resist the other. The use of play dough is excellent in promoting finger and hand actions. Other activities such as typing, needlework, piano playing, crafts, etc. are encouraged for arm, hand and finger exercise.

Exercises

ELBOW EXERCISES

Exercises 1-3 may be done either standing, sitting, or lying down. A graduated amount of weight can be held in the hand to increase strength as tolerated.

1. Support elbow on table, bend elbow, and raise hand toward shoulder.

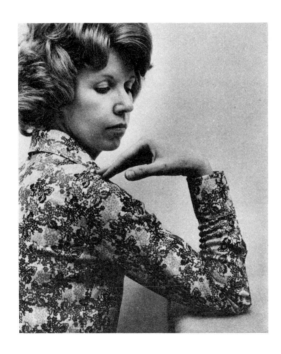

2. With elbow bent on table, lower hand.

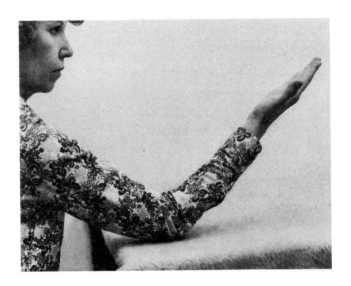

3. Support elbow on table with elbow bent. Turn palm up. Relax. Turn palm down. (this same action may be achieved by grasping a door knob and turning it as far as possible, first one direction, then the reverse.)

Exercises

WRIST EXERCISES

Sitting
1. With forearm resting on the table and palm flat, lift hand.

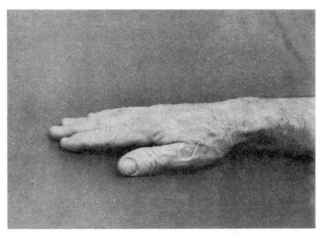

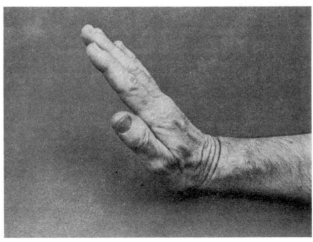

2. With palm down and forearm resting on table, turn wrist toward thumb side. Repeat, turning wrist toward little finger side.

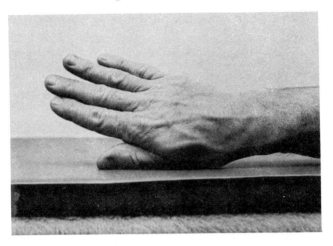

3. Rest forearm on table with hand resting on little finger side:

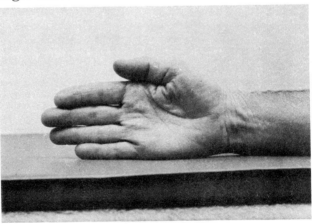

a) bend hand forward.

b) take hand backward.

c) lift hand toward thumb.

4. With forearm resting on table and wrist extended over the edge:

a) pull hand downward.

b) lift hand upward.

c) rotate wrist in all directions, using a circular motion. Reverse direction and repeat.

5. With both elbows bent and resting on a table, place hands together with fingers straight, then:

a) push toward left.

b) push toward right.

c) push toward little finger.

d) push toward thumb.

In this exercise the opposite hand can be used to assist or resist the action.

6. Same as #5 except fingers are interlocked. Repeat the above (a-d) motions and also perform a squeezing action.

TOE EXERCISES

Sitting

1. Bend and straighten toes.

2. Put turkish towel on floor and try to "grab and/or crumple" it with action of toes.
3. Place ball of foot over rung of chair and try to curl toes over rung.

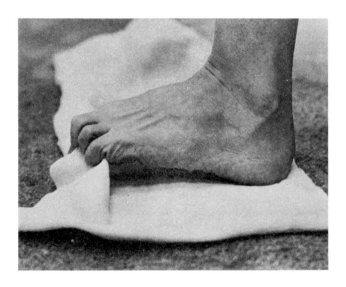

If joints can tolerate some weight bearing, you may stand and/or walk while shifting weight from outer border to inner border of feet, and from balls of feet back to heels.

HIP EXERCISES

Standing, support body by holding on to a firm surface such as a table or weighted chair.

    1. With knee straight, extend leg forward to fullest possible range. Hold and relax.

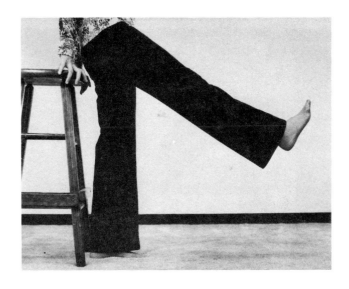

    2. With knee straight, move leg backward to fullest possible range. Hold and relax (do not bend trunk while doing this).

201

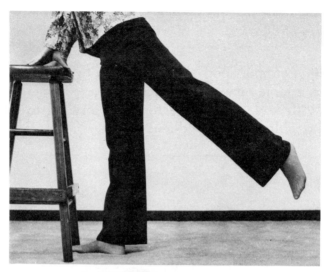

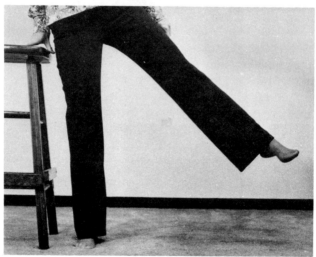

3. With knee straight, move leg out (away) to side. Hold. Move leg in to other leg.

Exercises

4. With knee straight, rotate leg in circular motion. Relax and repeat in opposite direction.
5. With knees straight, tighten low back muscles and pull leg up (this is called hip-hiking).
6. Place weight on opposite leg. With knee straight, turn foot, knee, and hip inward. Repeat, turning foot, knee, and hip outward.
7. Bend knee and bring it toward chest. Hold and then return it to the floor.

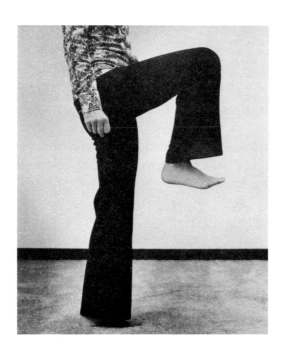

Exercises

8. Bend knee and perform "bicycling" action, emphasizing fullest range in all directions.

The above exercises are the simple hip joint range of motion movements and may be adapted for backlying, facelying, and sidelying position. You may require assistance in completing the range or may wish to add graduated resistance (with care) to strengthen the muscles.

KNEE EXERCISES

Sitting

1. Place a small firm cushion or towel roll under the thigh. Lift foot and straighten knee as far as possible. Hold, then bend knee and pull foot back. Hold and relax.
2. Both knees bent, turn knees away from each other, bringing soles of feet together. Repeat, turning knees toward one another, spreading feet apart.

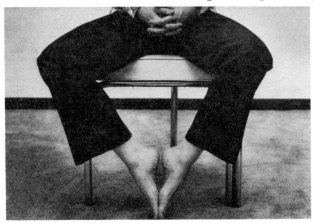

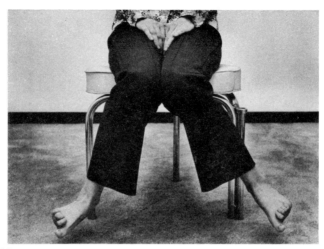

Backlying
    1. Bend knees with feet flat on the bed or floor. Lift foot by straightening the knee. Do alternately with right and left legs.

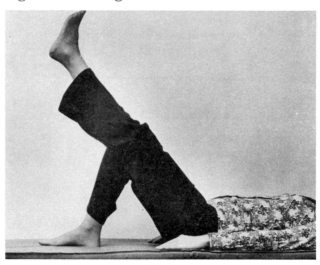

2. Place small towel roll under ankle, tighten thigh muscles and push knee toward bed (quad set).

Facelying

1. Place small pillow under abdomen, bend knee and draw foot backward toward buttock (do *not* lift hip from bed). Straighten knee and lower foot back to bed. May be done together or alternately.

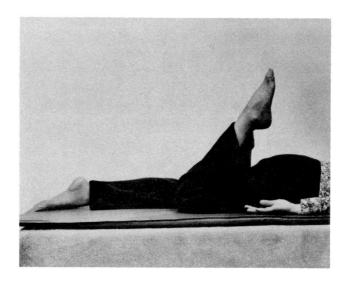

Standing

1. Practice stair climbing is an excellent knee extensor exercise if the joint can tolerate it.

Exercises

You may require assistance in completing the range of motion or you may wish to add graduated resistance to strengthen the muscles.

ANKLE EXERCISES

Sitting or Backlying
1. Bend ankle and raise toes up toward knee to fullest range possible. Hold and Relax.
2. Straighten ankle and point toes away from knee to fullest range possible. Hold and relax.
3. Bend ankle, raising toes up and in.
4. Bend ankle, raising toes up and out.
5. Straighten ankle, pointing toes down and in.
6. Straighten ankle, pointing toes down and out.
7. Rotate ankle in a circular motion. Repeat in opposite direction.
8. If joints can tolerate some weight bearing, you may stand and/or walk:
   a) on outer border of feet.
   b) on inner border of feet.
   c) on heels.
   d) on balls of feet.

Exercises

NECK EXERCISES

Sitting
1. Relax neck muscles and bend head forward (chin to chest). Slowly lift head up (sit tall), then backward slightly. Hold. Relax. Repeat.

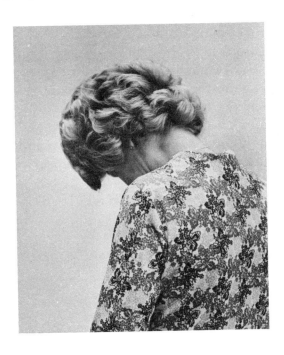

2. Direct chin toward shoulder, turning head to right (looking over shoulder). Hold. Relax. Repeat exercise in same manner to left.

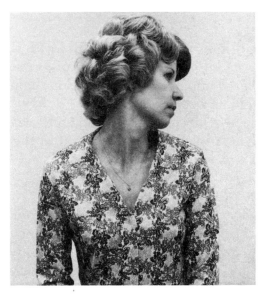

3. Looking straight ahead with chin slightly tucked, tip right ear toward right shoulder (do not lift shoulder). Hold. Relax and repeat exercise in same manner to left side.
4. Place fingertips behind neck with elbows pointing forward. Move elbows back slowly. Hold. Relax. This may be done standing. Keep chin slightly tucked in.
5. Sit with lower back against a wall. Gently press head back against the wall. Hold and relax. Do *not* tip head. This may also be done standing.
6. Loop a towel around your neck. Pull your chin in and at the same time pull forward on both ends of the towel. Resist the towel by pushing neck back. Relax and repeat. This may be done standing.

Exercises

Backlying
1. Lie with hips and knees bent and with a small flat pillow under your head. Gently press back of head downward into pillow, keeping chin slightly tucked in. Hold and relax. Repeat.
2. Lift head, chin on chest. Hold and relax. Repeat.
3. Turn head to right, then rotate it to the left side. Relax and repeat.

Facelying
1. On a firm surface with a small pillow under abdomen: Place your arms at your sides. Pinch shoulder blades together and raise your head and shoulders up about one inch. Turn head to the right, back to center, then to the left and back to the center. Do movements slowly and relax slowly. Repeat.

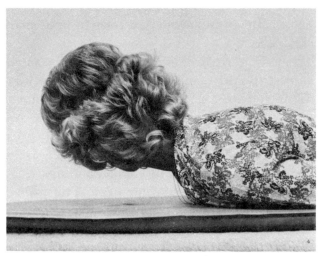

Glossary of Terms

ABDUCTION—Moving a limb away from the center of the body.

ACETABULUM—Cup-shaped cavity that the head of the femur (large bone of the thigh) fits into.

ACUPUNCTURE—Chinese practice of puncturing the body with needles to cure disease or relieve pain.

ADDUCTION—Moving a limb toward the center of the body.

ALIGNMENT—Proper positioning of the body parts in relation to one another.

AMBULATORY—Capable of walking about; not bedridden.

ANALGESIC—Pain relieving.

ARTHRITIS—Inflammation of joints.

ARTHRODESIS—Surgical immobilization (permanent) of a joint by fusion of the joint surfaces.

211

Glossary of Terms

ARTHROPLASTY—Plastic surgery of a joint.

ATROPHY—Wasting away of a body part or tissue.

AUTOSUGGESTION—A technique whereby one influences his own attitudes, behavior, or physical condition by mental processes other than conscious thought.

BIOFEEDBACK—The technique of making unconscious or involuntary body processes such as heartbeat or brain waves perceptible to the senses in order to manipulate them by conscious mental control.

BODY IMAGE—Mental picture each person has of his own body.

BUNION—Inflamed swelling of the small sac on the first joint of the big toe.

BURSA—A small sac filled with fluid, located between a tendon and a bone.

BURSITIS—Inflammation of a small sac filled with fluid which is located between a tendon and bone.

CALCIFICATION—Formation of deposits of calcium salts, rendering the affected area immovable.

CAPSULECTOMY—Removal of joint capsule.

CARTILAGE—Fibrous connective tissue.

CARTILAGENOUS/AMPHIARTHROSIS JOINT—A form of articulation permitting little motion; the surfaces of two bones are connected by fibrocartilage.

CATALYST—A separate agent that initiates action between two other forces.

Glossary of Terms

CERVICAL—Back part of the neck.

CLAW-TOE DEFORMITY—A deformity of the foot characterized by atrophy and distortion of the toes—usually the big toe—that results in a claw-like appearance.

CORTICOSTEROID—A compound produced naturally by a properly functioning adrenal gland.

CYLINDER GRASP—Holding an object parallel to the knuckles.

DECALCIFICATION—Decrease in or disappearance of calcium salts in tissue which cause immobilization.

DERMATITIS—Inflammation of the skin.

DIATHERMY—Generation of heat in tissues by electrical currents.

ELECTRODE—A conductor used to establish electrical contact with a nonmetallic part of a circuit.

EXTENSION—Moving into a straight position.

FEMORAL HEAD—Top part of femur or thigh bone.

FIBROCARTILAGE—A type of connective tissue containing many fibers which serve to stabilize it and prevent movement.

FIBROSITIS—Inflammation of fibrous tissue of the body, marked by pain and stiffness.

FIBROUS/SYNARTHROSES JOINT—A form of articulation in which the bones are united by continuous intervening fibrous tissue.

Glossary of Terms

FLEXION—Bending.

FLEXURE CONTRACTION—Inability to straighten joint caused by shortening of muscle.

HAMSTRINGS—Tendons in back of knee.

HEMOGLOBIN—Protein occurring in red blood cells which carries oxygen and contains iron.

HYALINE CARTILAGE—Glassy, nearly transparent connective tissue.

HYDROCOLLATOR PACK—A pack of solid material which becomes a gel when soaked in water; used to apply heat or cold to body parts.

HYPERVITAMINOSIS—Condition due to excess of vitamins.

HYPOCHRONDRIA—Condition wherein a person often centers on imaginery physical ailments; extreme depression of mind or spirits.

ISOMETRIC EXERCISE—Exercise involving great amount of muscle contraction, but no joint motion. Opposing muscles are contracted with little shortening but great increase in tone of muscle fibers involved.

JACOBSON'S PROGRESSIVE RELAXATION EXERCISES—a system of exercises in which the patient is taught to distinguish between relaxed and contracted muscles. This is accomplished by having the patient contract a muscle or group of muscles to its fullest extent and then fully relax it.

JOINT—Place where two body parts are joined.

Glossary of Terms

KYPHOSIS—Forward curvature of the upper spine, i.e., humpback.

LIBIDO—Sexual drive.

LIGAMENT—Tough band of tissue connecting bones or supporting organs in place.

LORDOSIS—Exaggerated forward curvature of the lower spine.

LUMBAR—Lower back.

METABOLISM—Process by which energy is made available to the body.

MODALITY—A therapeutic measure or agency, such as heat or cold, used in physical therapy.

MUSCULOSKELETAL—Involving both musculature and skeleton.

MYOSITIS—Inflammation of a voluntary muscle.

OCCUPATIONAL THERAPY—Therapy by means of activity, as in creative activity for rehabilitation.

OSTEOMYELITIS—Inflammation of bone.

OSTEONECROSIS—Death of bone.

OSTEOPHYTES—Bony outgrowths caused by disease.

OSTEOPOROSIS—Thinning of the bones.

OSTEOTOMY—Surgical cutting of bone.

PHLEBITIS—Inflammation of a vein.

215

Glossary of Terms

PHYSICAL THERAPY—Treatment of a disease by mechanical or physical means such as heat, light, massage, regulated exercise, water.

PHYSIOLOGICAL—Pertaining to the activities and functions of the body.

PLANTAR NERVE—Nerve in sole of foot.

POLYARTERITIS (Nordosa)—Inflammation of arteries.

PROSTHESES—An artificial device to replace a missing part of the body.

PURINE—Substance from which uric acid compounds are formed.

QUADRICEPS MUSCLES—Large muscles in front part of thighs.

RAYNAUD'S DISEASE—A disorder of the blood vessels characterized by intermittent attacks of pallor, cold, and loss of sensation in the extremities.

ROTATION—Circular movement around a fixed point.

SCOLIOSIS—An appreciable lateral deviation in the normally straight vertical line of the spine.

SEDIMENTATION RATE—Rate of sinking of red blood cells in measured amount of blood.

SELF-ESTEEM—Confidence and satisfaction in oneself.

SERUM PROTEINS—Proteins found in clear part of blood when blood components are separated into serum and clotted material.

Glossary of Terms

SUPINATION—Rotation of arm so that palm faces upward.

SYNOVECTOMY—Removal of the lining of the capsule of a joint.

SYNOVIAL FLUID—Transparent lubricating fluid secreted by synovial membrane; resembles white of an egg.

SYNOVIAL MEMBRANE—Membrane which secretes synovial fluid; found in bursae, joint cavities, and tendon sheaths.

SYNOVIAL/DIARTHRODIAL JOINT—A joint composed of two different joint surfaces which are surrounded by synovial fluid.

TARSAL TUNNEL SYNDROME—Pressure on nerve in center of foot, can cause pain, lack of sensation, and/or other symptoms such as tingling.

TENDON—Tough cord or band of connective tissue that unites a muscle with some other part.

TENOTOMY—Cutting of a tendon.

THERAPEUTIC—Treatment which attempts to relieve a disease or condition.

TRACTION—Pulling force exerted on skeleton by a special device.

TRANSCUTANEOUS NERVE STIMULATION (TNS)—A technique for interrupting messages to the brain while they are in the nerve pathways en route from the site of stimulation to the brain. A unit is attached to the patient's waist and electrodes running from it are

217

attached to various sites along the nerve pathways. A low intensity electrical current is generated by the unit and transmitted via the electrodes. This electrical stimulation blocks transmission of message to the brain.

TRICEPS—Large muscle along the back of the upper arm.

ULNAR DEVIATION—Displacement of the hand in the direction of the little finger.

ULTRASOUND—Vibrations with the same physical nature as sound but with frequencies above the range of human hearing; sometimes used to treat musculo-skeletal disorders.

URIC ACID—Acid formed by urine; excess is a symptom of gout.

VALGUS DEFORMITY—A type of deformity in which the body part is bent outward from the center of the body.

VERTEBRA—Bone of the spinal column.

WRY NECK—Contraction of the neck muscles which produces twisting of the neck.

Appendix

DISTRIBUTORS AND MANUFACTURERS OF REHABILI-
TATION AIDS AND EQUIPMENT

Be. O.K. Sales Co.
Box 32
Brookfield, Illinois 60513

Cleo Living Aids
3957 Mayfield Road
Cleveland, Ohio 44121

Everest & Jennings
1803 Pontius Avenue
Los Angeles, California 90025

Fred Sammons, Inc.
Box 32
Brookfield, Illinois 60513

G.E. Miller, Inc.
484 Broadway
Yonkers, N.Y. 10705

Personal Health Services, Inc.
4800 Oakland Street, Suite G
Denver, Colorado 80239

J.A. Preston Corporation
71 Fifth Avenue South
New York, N.Y. 10003

Rehab Aids
5913 S.W. 8th Street
Miami, Florida 33144

Rehabilitation Equipment, Inc.
175 East 83rd Street
New York, N.Y. 10028

Rehabilitation Products
American Hospital Supply Corp.
2020 Ridge Avenue
Evanston, Illinois 60201

Scully Walton
505 East 116th Street
New York, N.Y. 10023

Winco Products, Winfield Co., Inc.
3062-46th Avenue
St. Petersburg, Florida 33714

CLOTHING

Fashion-Able
Rocky Hill, New Jersey 08553

Appendix

"Flexible Fashions"— a brochure available from
U.S. Dept. HEW, Public Health Service
Publication #1814
Superintendent of Documents
U.S. Printing Office
Washington, D.C. 20402   Cost: 20¢

Talon, Inc.
"Shu-lok" Division
43 East 51st Street
New York, N.Y. 10022

Vocational Guidance and Rehabilitation Services
2239 East 55th Street
Cleveland, Ohio 44103

RECREATION

American Association for Health, Physical Education
and Recreation
Program for the Handicapped
1201 16th Street N.W.
Washington, D.C. 20036

National Parks and Forestry
Survey by the President's Committee on the
Unemployment of the Handicapped
Washington, D.C. 20210

Appendix

National Recreation and Park Association and National
Therapeutic Recreation Society
1700 Pennsylvania Ave. N.W.
Washington, D.C. 20006
1601 No. Kent Street
Arlington, Virginia 22209

"Your Garden and Your Rheumatism," by C.B. Heald,
a brochure available from Canadian Arthritis and
Rheumatism Society
45 Charles Street East
Toronto 5, Canada   Cost: 30¢

INFORMATION ON ARTHRITIS

American Rheumatism Association
1212 Avenue of the Americas
New York, N.Y. 10036

Arthritis Foundation
3400 Peachtree Road
Atlanta, Georgia 30326

National Institutes of Arthritis and Metabolic Diseases
Bethesda, Maryland 20014

Index

223

Index

Index

Laundry tasks, 68-69
Leukeran, 87
Librium, 89
Lifting, 60-62
Limp, 47
Lordosis, 50

Massage, 34-35
Meal preparation, 69-72
Meals on Wheels, 118-19
Medications for treatment of
    arthritis, 79-90, 137-38
Medrol, 86
Methotrexate, 87
Mexican clinics, 142
Minimum daily requirements, 114-15
Mixing, hand, 70-71
Motrin, 84-85, 158
Muscle re-education, 101-102
Muscle relaxants, 89
Music, 149

Nalfon, 84-85
Naprosyn, 84-85
Nature walks, 150
Neck
    exercises for the, 208-210
    problems of the, 49
Norflex, 89
Nurses, public health, 125-26
Nutrition, 113-121

Occupational therapist, 42
Osteoarthritis, 8-12, 104, 105
Osteoporosis, 120, 143
Osteotomy, 106-7
Oxalid, 82

Pain
    control of, 91-103
    in osteoarthritis, 11
Paraffin bath, hot, 37-38
Parafon, 89
Passive exercise, 22-23
Patient, responsibilities of, 127-28
Penicillamine, 89
Phone grip, 74
Physical therapist, 42

Physical therapy, 27-40, 126-27
Plaquenil, 82
Playing cards, 75
Pool exercises, 159-67
    benefits of, 154-56
    restrictions, 158-59
Positioning, correct, 16-20
Posture, correct, 16-18, 20
Prednisone, 86
Primary gout, 13-14
Primary osteoarthritis, 10
Propoxyphene, 88
Prostheses, 109-110
Psychological counseling, 111
Psychosocial effects of arthritis, 129-38, 140
Purinethol, 87

Radiation, 32-33
Range of motion exercises, 23
Raynaud's Disease, 101
Reading, 75
Relaxation in water, 155-56
Relaxation training, 98-101
Resistive exercise, 23
Rest, 20-21
Rest-exercise program, 21-26
Rheumatic diseases, 3-4
Rheumatoid arthritis, 4-8, 104-5, 119-20
Robaxin, 89

Salicylates, 80-81
Salvage surgery, 105, 106
Sayre traction, 36, 49-50
Scissors, 75
Scoliosis, 50
Secondary gout, 14
Secondary osteoarthritis, 10
Self-esteem, loss of, 132
Sexuality, 136-37
Shoes, 44
Shoulder exercises, 163-64, 173-74, 177-86
Side effects of medications, 137-38
Sitting, 17-18
Skin temperature, increasing, 100-101
Social status, loss of, 135-36

225

Index